The Tibetan Book of Health

MENLA SORIG SERIES

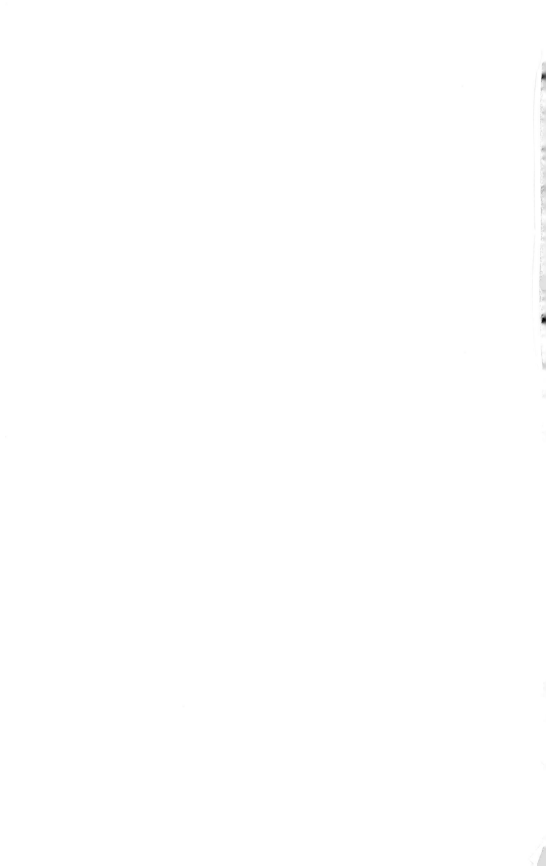

The Tibetan Book of Health

Sowa Rigpa, the Science of Healing

DR. NIDA CHENAGTSANG

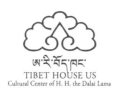

ཨ་རི་བོད་ཁང་
TIBET HOUSE US
Cultural Center of H. H. the Dalai Lama

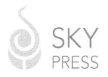

SKY
PRESS

Copublished by:

Tibet House US
22 West 15th Street
New York, NY 10011
www.tibethouse.us

Sky Press
3640 SE Washington Street
Portland, OR 97214
www.skypressbooks.com

Distributed internationally in the English language by Sky Press

Library of Congress Control Number: 2017936924

ISBN 978-0-9977319-4-1

27 26 25 24 23 22 21 20 19 18 17   1 2 3 4 5 6 7 8 9

Second English Edition
Printed in the United States of America, the United Kingdom, and Australia
on acid-free paper

EDITORS: Jacqueline Yu, Dr. Anastazja Holečko
COEDITOR: Scott Mist, PhD
MANUSCRIPT EDITOR: Leslie Kriesel

INTERIOR DESIGN: William Meyers
COVER DESIGN: Milenda Nan Ok Lee
COVER IMAGE: robertharding / Alamy Stock Photo

Interior images courtesy of Sorig Khang International

The medical information in this book is provided without any representations or
warranties, expressed or implied. You must not rely on the information in this book
as an alternative to medical advice from your doctor or other professional health-care
provider. If you think you may be suffering from any medical condition, you should
seek immediate medical attention.

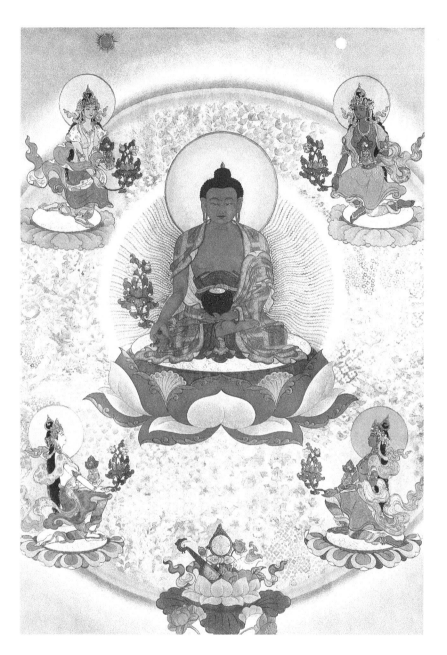

Sangye Menla—The Medicine Buddha

Contents

Foreword

Robert A. F. Thurman

I AM HONORED to write a foreword for Dr. Nida's *Tibetan Book of Health*. He is a great spiritual teacher, an excellent Tibetan doctor, and a good friend. For me, he has brought to life the amazing spiritual, scientific, and medical teachings of the great Yuthok Yönten Gönpo the younger (1126–1202) in this present very difficult, though still promising, world era.

Shakyamuni, the Buddha (ca. sixth century B.C.E.), has been the champion of human scientists from his time up to now. This may surprise you, because he is mainly known as the founder of the "world religion" called Buddhism. Since we categorize religion as the opposite of science, it seems odd to hear that he was a scientist, and supreme among them. But it is very easily reasoned that he did fully understand body, mind, and the world, in both their relative and ultimate natures, and that he discovered, to our great relief, that the reality in which we exist is fundamentally just fine for everyone. Wherever we are is perfectly all right, supportive and fulfilling, *if we understand it*—our habitual suffering within it comes only from our *ignorance* of its nature, our lack of understanding.

Thus the job of anyone who does understand it all, and therefore has found fulfillment and happiness, is to try to educate others who suffer due to their misunderstanding, to help them come to understand the positive reality for themselves.

"Science" is defined as the organized body of knowledge and empirical method that aims to discover the exact nature of reality, and a real "scientist" is a knower of at least some aspects of such reality and a practitioner of the methods to improve that knowledge. In recent centuries, "reality" has become defined as "physical" or "material," so many would define modern science as inescapably grounded in a worldview of materialism. The "mental," as the opposite of the material, has been defined out of existence, and mental phenomena are supposed to be systematically reduced to manifestations of material processes.

But the definition of science as materialism is not itself the result of a scientific discovery. No one has ever discovered the nothing that is supposed to be the absence of the mental, anything other than the material. When you look for a mental object and don't find it as a material object, you have not failed to find a mental object, you have simply not found your conception of it as a material object. Your act of not finding it is itself actually a mental process, but you don't notice it as that, because you're not looking for it.

Materialist science is imprisoned by a philosophical mix-up. Scientists need to set themselves free by learning from the great scientists of India and Tibet how to own up to the fact that they are beings who have minds, spirits, and even souls—not as some sort of mystical entities, but as rationally explorable and experientially understandable processes. These processes are extremely subtle, and to learn about them, understand them, and so master them requires a new kind of advanced education and training of one's own emotional, intellectual, and mental abilities.

The Buddha, and millions of his successors in his scientific tradition that still thrives all over the world after at least 2,600 years, was a champion philosopher, and therefore was able to be a champion scientist. He rejected the religious beliefs and dogmas of his day and decided that the good and appropriate life would have to be based on realistic knowledge of its true nature. He was not so naïve as to proceed to investigate the world in denial of the existence of his mind. He realized that, though subtle and elusive, it was the most important function of his body-mind complex, regulating its quality of life and determining its experiences and its reactions.

After a youth devoted to study and pleasure within the conventional culture of his era, he departed on his quest for the deepest knowledge, and after six years of strenuous exploration of body, mind, and universe, he experienced the reality he was looking for. He experienced it fully and completely, and so came to be called "a buddha," perfectly enlightened. His report back on what he found has puzzled people ever since. Instead of handing out a formula that contained all answers, he said that real reality cannot be captured in verbal or mathematical formulae; it is way too deep, vast, and complex to be so reduced. Verbal and mathematical formulations are essential, as they provide direction for the systematic experiential explorations required for ultimate discovery. Like modern science in its method aspect, he privileged experience over theory, acknowledging the limitations of theory and assuring human beings of the potentially unlimited reach of well-cultivated and intensely focused experience.

I go into this only enough to suggest that what the Buddha called the "inner science" that enabled him and his successors to discover the reality of both the physical and the mental, coarse and subtle, aspects of life and the world, is the realistic understanding of reality itself. The claim is that a perfectly enlightened Buddha is a human being who expands her or his intelligence and opens her or his experiential instruments enough to become fully aware of the realities of the self, of the processes of life and death, and of the exact nature of physical reality—though any description of such realities relying on conventional communicative systems will inevitably fall short of capturing their inconceivably amazing nature. The only general encouragement given us is that reality itself is just wonderful. It is freedom, it is fulfillment, it is within us as the real happiness we are constantly searching for elsewhere.

The corollary of this claim is that among the realities understood by such a scientist is the reality of the human intelligence: its infinite expandability, its ability to understand whatever it focuses on methodically with supercritical analysis and supernormal concentration, and its potential to enable any human being to become a perfect buddha through a conscious evolutionary process of prolonged education and training.

The further corollary of this second claim is the third claim that the foremost "outer science" developed by the Buddha and his successors— the medical science, the science and arts of healing—is based on realistic knowledge of the human body and mind and of the nature of this planet to which the human being is so well adapted. It is not just a premodern, backward, nonscientific system, developed by ancient people who didn't have all our modern equipment and theories. To the contrary—and modern psychology ("inner science") is still very much in the dark about how people's minds really work and the mind-body interrelationship, due to its determination to join the material sciences and its stubborn insistence that there is no mind. Denying its own subject matter, psyche or mind, it asserts that mental states are reducible to chemicals and physical neurological mechanisms. Likewise, modern medical science is trapped in a disease-focused approach, relying mainly on surgery and drugs, and has lost touch with the reality of health and sickness that comes from our high-tech, antinatural, high-stress industrial environment.

There has been quite a bit of public health progress in recent centuries, mainly due to measures such as washing hands, inoculations, sanitation systems, somewhat improved birthing techniques, refinement of surgical skills and procedures, and so on. Life expectancy has increased in certain segments of global society. However, we are all still victims of our backward material cultures' inability to control population growth; the pollution of soil, water, and air; the corporate commercialization of agriculture and food production, processing, and delivery; drug production; and hospital care, all unchecked by corporation-captured regulatory agencies. Our physicians themselves suffer from a dehumanizing medical school curriculum that does not teach the Hippocratic healing principles except by osmosis, disdains knowledge of nutrition, and socializes and trains the students to staff the corporate-dominated drugs-and-surgery intervention industries. We, the patients, beneficiaries sometimes and victims sometimes, are trained to place our faith in this system.

In this situation, *The Tibetan Book of Health* comes as a breath of fresh air. It is the gift of scientifically as well as spiritually enlightened healers, who not only understand what ails us but also know how to help us understand ourselves and become more conscious about our own health and how to sustain it. First priority for the enlightened healer physicians is awakening us patients to the way our own body-mind complex works in terms we can easily understand. The whole point is to expand our vision of ourselves as beings in a nature that is luckily more beneficial than harmful, especially if we understand how it works.

Dr. Nida is a master of the spiritual, mental, or "inner" science that is the basis of the healing science. He is widely loved and respected in his homeland in Amdo province of northeast ethnic Tibet (present-day Qinghai province of China). He also is highly skilled and experienced in administering healing to mind and body of many patients all over the world, not only in Tibet but also in the Russias, especially the Buddhist republics;

Mongolia; China; Nepal; India—all countries where the Tibetan medicine tradition is honored and widely used—and even in Europe, where there is a high degree of interest in the tradition. He has become especially renowned for reviving in clinical practice the practice of what are called the "external therapies," such as massage, cupping, tapping, acupuncture, etc. He presents in this *Book of Health* the good news of the tradition's view of life as encouragingly manageable, as well as information that practitioner and patient can use in improving their lives.

I am particularly happy to inaugurate this series of Menla Sorig Series texts in collaboration with Sky Press, the publishing house for Dr Nida's organization, Sorig Khang International (SKI), since Menla and SKI share the intention to bring Tibetan Medicine into a more public light around the world. Sowa Rigpa is not only a theory, but living medical tradition. The Mahasukha Spa at Menla Mountain Retreat and Spa Resort is the first spa in the United States that is built upon the principles of Sowa Rigpa and offers therapies in the various healing methods described in this book.

The book is meant to serve as the foundation of Dr. Nida's teaching of his many students around the world. I am very impressed by the editor, Jacqueline Yu, startled and delighted to read her account of the experience of learning from Dr. Nida the teachings recorded in this book:

> I still remembered his teachings clearly, as every word spoken was an awakening process and everything suddenly became crystal clear to me. It was to be the start of my continual learning journey in the vast map of *Sowa Rigpa,* or traditional Tibetan medicine. And it is indeed my good fortune to study with a teacher who is able to impart such profundity in a very clear and simple way, mostly with a good measure of humor thrown in.

When I was first seriously studying Tibetan Buddhism, my teacher, the Venerable Geshe Wangyal, read to me the *Friendly Letter* written by the great Nāgārjuna, giving a summary of the whole Buddhist reality and path. I had the very experience—"every word spoken was an awakening process and everything suddenly became crystal clear to me"—that Ms. Yu describes, and I consider this to be an unusual and precious mark of a great teaching and a great teacher. I welcome all readers who want to enjoy a healthy life, and also to help others enjoy the same.

With my thanks to Dr. Nida first of all, and to those of his students whom I know and admire, Dr. Tam Nguyen, Dr. Anastazja Holečko, Eric Rosenbush, Jacqueline Yu, and Christiana Polites.

Robert A. F. Thurman
Jey Tsong Khapa Professor of Indo-Tibetan Buddhist Studies
Columbia University
President, Tibet House US
Co-Founder, Menla Retreat and Spa Resort

Preface

TRADITIONAL Tibetan Medicine, known as Sowa Rigpa, the "Science of Healing," is one of the oldest healing traditions in existence, yet it remains fully alive and intact today. A truly holistic system of medicine that approaches the health of an individual at the levels of the physical body, energy, and mind, it has the fourfold aim of preventing illness, curing illness, extending life, and cultivating happiness. Through the tireless work, writing, and teaching activities of Dr. Nida Chenagtsang we have the good fortune of having a window into this vast tradition, previously accessible only to those native to the lands of Sowa Rigpa, including Tibet, neighboring Himalayan regions, and Mongolia. Dr. Nida's international nonprofit foundation, Sorig Khang International (www.sorig.net), has branch centers in more than forty countries worldwide with courses of study happening year-round in dozens of languages. SKY Press was founded in 2016 to help make the valuable material taught at these centers available to the general public so that it may reach a wider audience and benefit not only students and practitioners of Sowa Rigpa but anyone seeking health, balance, and happiness in life.

One of Dr. Nida's great gifts as a teacher is his ability to teach sophisticated subjects, both medical and spiritual (which in Sowa Rigpa are never separate), in a manner that can inspire and benefit anyone, from the beginning student to the advanced practitioner. His words are simple, clear, and direct, yet they contain many layers of meaning that unfold as one's own understanding deepens and matures with time and experience. *The Tibetan Book of Health* is one such teaching. It offers a complete overview of the theory and practice of Tibetan medicine in language that is accessible to those with no prior exposure to the subject, but at the same time it may serve as a reference for both students and practitioners of Sowa Rigpa as it contains a wealth of information that can be contemplated and returned to again and again.

Special thanks to Jacqueline Yu for her work in editing and compiling this book and for the support of Anastazja Holečko. From Tibet House Publications, I sincerely thank William Meyers for laying out the interior pages of this book and Milenda Lee for the beautiful cover design, and I especially thank Professor Robert Thurman for being the inspiration behind this collaboration. Professor Thurman and Dr. Nida have much in common, not only in the depth and breadth of their knowledge, but also in their limitless and bubbling enthusiasm for the subjects to which they have dedicated their lives, and the long-term vision of the positive role that Sowa Rigpa will play in the coming times. Their vision and enthusiasm is contagious—in their presence I have the feeling that there is nothing that is impossible, the sky is the limit. When they teach side by side at Menla Mountain Retreat Center their friendship, the deep respect that they share for each other's knowledge and work, and their love of this medicine permeates the whole environment. So it is with the utmost joy that we present this book, the first in what I hope will be many future collaborations between Tibet House Publications and SKY Press on Sowa Rigpa, and a deep and enduring friendship.

Christiana Polites
SKY Press
February 20th, 2017
Portland, Oregon
www.skypressbooks.com

Editor's Note

How amazing it is to read on Tibetan medicine!
How awe-inspiring it is to learn Tibetan medicine!
How wonderful it is to practice Tibetan medicine!

I first came across Tibetan medicine through Dr. Yeshe Dhonden's book *Health Through Balance* and find the world of Tibetan medicine so fascinating. In 2008, I invited Dr. Nida Chenagtsang to teach in Singapore. Thus began my Tibetan medical studies, starting with Mantra Healing and *Kunye*, traditional Tibetan massage. I still remembered his teachings clearly, as every word spoken was an awakening process and everything suddenly became crystal clear to me. It was to be the start of my continual learning journey in the vast map of *Sowa Rigpa,* or traditional Tibetan medicine. And it is indeed my good fortune to study with a teacher who is able to impart such profundity in a very clear and simple way, mostly with a good measure of humor thrown in.

When Dr. Nida asked me to edit his new book on Tibetan medicine, I was both honored and grateful to be a part of this great project. The first part of this book contains basic explanations about Sowa Rigpa and its philosophy. It comprises a summary of Dr. Nida's medical teachings and of his textbook *Root Tantra*, used in the International Academy for

Traditional Tibetan Medicine (IATTM)'s education programs. A book like this is so important to provide a clear, basic understanding of the theory and structure of Tibetan medicine and also its practical value. It will be beneficial for both the general public as well as serious students of Sowa Rigpa. And I hope that just as I was inspired, you will be inspired to learn more and also benefit from it immeasurably.

No book would be possible without all the people involved. Of course, thanks to Dr. Nida first and foremost for imparting this profound knowledge and for sharing unreservedly. And to Scott Mist for the many hours working on the first editorial part. To Dr. Anastazja Holečko for helping to put the whole book together! And finally to all who contributed in one way or another, I offer my sincere gratitude.

Jacqueline Yu
Yuthok Nyingthig Guru Yoga Retreat,
Singapore

The Tibetan Book of Health

Introduction

IN TIBET, in the eighth century C.E., there was a man who lived 125 years and achieved the rainbow body—the expression of complete spiritual realization—along with his wife and his dog. This man was Yuthok Yönten Gönpo, the Elder (708–833), the father of traditional Tibetan medicine, a great teacher of health, who attained the spiritual realization of the body, energy, and mind.[1]

However, he left a question unresolved. How did he live for so long and attain so many extraordinary accomplishments?

Thanks to his enormous compassion, we can find within his writings the answers to these questions, which can be used either for the improvement of our health or for the benefit of all sentient beings. All his knowledge is still available to us. Through an unbroken lineage, the work of many traditional Tibetan medicine teachers, doctors, practitioners, and training institutions, this ancient healing science, otherwise known as *Sowa Rigpa*, is

---

[1] He attained such a realization, which was demonstrated through his achievement of the rainbow body, of which there are many levels; Yuthok achieved the complete rainbow body. His body dissolved into light and rainbows, natural sounds were heard, the earth moved, five colored lights were seen, there was a clear sky, and it rained flowers for three months; all these are the signs of the highest realization.

spreading its wings and finding a new audience in many parts of the world. Many people and patients are benefiting from the practices of *Sowa Rigpa*.

This "Tibetan book of health" is only a small map of one portion of the great wisdom of Yuthok! It should be understood as an introduction to the foundations of Sowa Rigpa. I hope to deepen this journey through the various disciplines comprised by this ancient science of healing. And I hope this book will bring benefits to all who read it and apply the advice it contains.

Sorig Khang International (SKI), formerly known as the International Academy for Traditional Tibetan Medicine (IATTM), is encouraging small-scale research work from practitioners worldwide. Even individual case studies or small collections of case reports are, when properly conducted and documented, a valuable source of scientific information. They can be published in scientific journals and thereby help to further the reputation and increase the credibility of Sowa Rigpa. Adopting accepted methods of scientific research requires Sowa Rigpa practitioners to implement certain methodologies into their practice. Standardization, quality control, and documentation are some of these rather rigid aspects. This requires a certain change in thinking—from the patient-centered individual approach of Sowa Rigpa to the statistical, impersonal approach of modern science. The practitioner working with Sowa Rigpa in the modern environment has to bridge both worlds, traditional and modern scientific. In this way tradition can learn from modern techniques and even gain an insight into the mechanisms of its own methods. Likewise, the modern doctor or scientist from a conventional academic background can take inspiration from time-tested traditional knowledge to broaden their horizons. The future of Sowa Rigpa lies in this bridging effort, through which we can serve humanity far into the future.

Dr. Nida Chenagtsang
Rome, Italy, 2014

1

The Healing Garden

A Brief Introduction

TRADITIONAL Tibetan Medicine (TTM) or *Sowa Rigpa* (Tib. *gso ba rig pa*) has an ancient origin and through an unbroken lineage is available to us in our time. *Sowa* is translated as "Healing" and *Rigpa* as "Science," i.e., Healing Science. Another meaning of *Sowa Rigpa* is "Nourishment of Awareness," with *Sowa* translated as "Nourishment" and *Rigpa* as "Awareness."

At the heart of this medical system is a deep connection with nature. One can learn a great deal through the observation of nature, and it permeates Sowa Rigpa. Metaphors from nature are used to categorize, memorize, and explain the various aspects of medicine.

There are 99 trees of knowledge in the arboreal metaphor commonly known as the Trees of Tibetan Medicine. These function as a summary, as well as a detailed and methodical learning aid whereby the core content of Tibetan medical knowledge is portrayed in the form of branching trees, with subtopics as branches, stems, and leaves. As in an abundant garden, one who is dedicated to studying this medicine will move between roots, stems, branches, leaves, flowers, and fruits, learning as much as possible about each part.

The human structure, physically and mentally, can also be compared to nature and the physiology of a tree. The roots are like the brain; the trunk is the body that, if well nourished, grows in a healthy and lush way; the branches and leaves are like the body tissues; the fruits are comparable to what we do in our life. If we do good deeds, we have good health; conversely, if we do not take care of our body and mind, like a plant without water, good air, and fertile land, they will not produce fruit. The Tibetan physician, like a good gardener with an abundance of knowledge, seeks to heal and prevent illnesses in every part of the tree.

Sowa Rigpa emphasizes the interdependent relationship between human health and nature. Therefore the Tibetan physician finds that it is not a coincidence that with increasing pollution and adulteration of food products, there has been an increased incidence of allergic disorders, food intolerance, and heart and respiratory diseases. Tibetan herbal formulas such as Sedru 5 (based on pomegranate) and Lishi 6 (based on clove) can be very beneficial for allergies and prevent respiratory problems respectively. External therapies like moxibustion, cupping, and even mantras can also help address these issues.

Sowa Rigpa is a complete system of healing that, due to interaction with various cultural elements, has become a unique science different from other medical systems. Within Sowa Rigpa we can find subject matter related to both psychological and energetic aspects, which Western biomedicine has been exploring only recently. Moreover, Sowa Rigpa includes a well-developed and abundant philosophical system, a structure of subtle anatomy, and a spiritual practice including knowledge of embryology, anatomy, physiology, pathology, diagnosis, pharmacopoeia, and external therapies, which is still barely known in the West.

Attention is directed not just to sick people but also to people seeking to maintain their health. The main aim of this medicine is the prevention of imbalance, the maintenance of physical, mental, and energetic health. When this is not possible, because an imbalance or disorder has led to the emergence of a disease, then the next aim is to find a cure. For this reason, the treatment offered by a Tibetan physician is meant not only to cure a disease but also to teach the patient how to live in balance with this mandala that spans from the most inner and subtle energetics to the external environment.

Sowa Rigpa is thus a medical science that looks at the human being as a whole, not in a piecemeal way commonly found in the modern clinic, paying attention to the interconnections that exist within us, between us and everything that surrounds us, and all sentient beings and nature. Thus if we pollute the Earth and its waters, destroy forests and other natural habitats, we will experience the health consequences, which is unfortunately already happening.

If we are aware that we are affected by events beyond the physical body, energy, and mind, which can have an important role in our health or lead to the appearance of problems or diseases, then the lure of traditional Tibetan medicine becomes obvious. The results obtained from Sowa Rigpa practice over the centuries prove its effectiveness in maintaining health.

Tibetan medicine, like much of Tibetan culture, is infused with terminology and concepts that derive from Buddhism. But it is important to

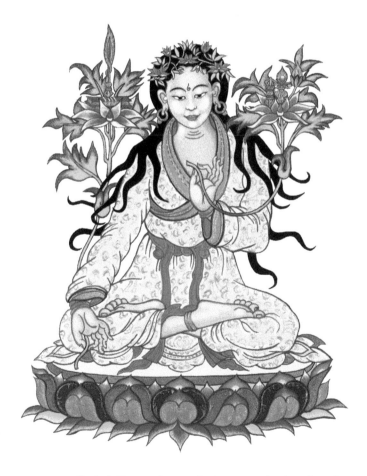

FIG. 1. Yuthok Yönten Gönpo the Younger, the founder of Tibetan medicine

understand that Sowa Rigpa is not itself a Buddhist practice. It is rather a traditional medicine that can benefit all, Tibetans and non-Tibetans, Buddhists and non-Buddhists. The task of the Tibetan doctor is to treat everyone. This is reflected in the words of Yuthok Yönten Gönpo, the Younger (1126–1201),[1] the father of Sowa Rigpa, who in the twelfth century wrote: "My desire is that Tibetan medicine can spread like the infinite expanse of the sky, for the benefit of all sentient beings."

---

[1] There are two Yuthok Yönten Gönpos: the Elder, in the eighth century, and the Younger, in the twelfth century, a famous descendant of the previous Yuthok. Both are considered the father of Tibetan medicine, as the elder wrote the first medical texts and the younger reorganized and rewrote these texts, the *Four Tantras* and other well-known works still used by students and doctors to the present day.

2

The Medicine Buddha Mandala
and Four Tantras

THIS NATURAL and perfect science of health was born from the primordial wisdom of Yuthok, a manifestation in human form of the Medicine Buddha.[1] In this chapter we will begin to explore his teachings, and in doing so introduce many new terms and concepts. Many of these are explored later on, while some of them are beyond the scope of this book.

The Medicine Buddha Mandala is a graphical representation of Yuthok's insight. A mandala[2] is a symbol of the perfect balance of all five elements. Everything inside is equivalent to everything outside. It is formed by a center and four directions. It can express the five Wisdoms (the five positive aspects of our mind), the five Dhyani Buddhas (Five Family Buddhas representing the five qualities of the Buddha), the five Dakinis (female enlightened beings portrayed as consorts of the male buddhas), etc. Fundamentally, however, the mandala represents the five elements—space,

---

[1] In Tibetan he is known as SANGYE MENLA: SANG (awake) GYE (developed of five wisdoms) MEN (medicine) LA (Guru).

[2] Mandala (Sanskrit: *maṇḍala*, "circle")—the Sanskrit root *man* means mind, which is similar to the Latin word *mens*. It is a spiritual and ritual symbol in Hinduism and Buddhism, representing the universe, consisting of five elements. One element is at the center and the remaining four are in different directions.

wind, fire, water, and earth—indicated by blue, green, red, white, and yellow respectively.

The Mandala of the Medicine Buddha is called Tanadug (in Tib. *lta na sdug*), which means town or enchanted garden. The central part is blue, north is green, east is white, west is red, and south is yellow.

In the introductory chapter of his medical works, Yuthok Yönten Gön-po describes this enchanted garden and the way the "Four Tantras" were born. The *Four Tantras* or *Gyud Shi* (Tib. *rgyud bzhi*) is the fundamental Tibetan medical text comprising four volumes. The following journey through Tanadug is rewritten from the first and second chapter of *The*

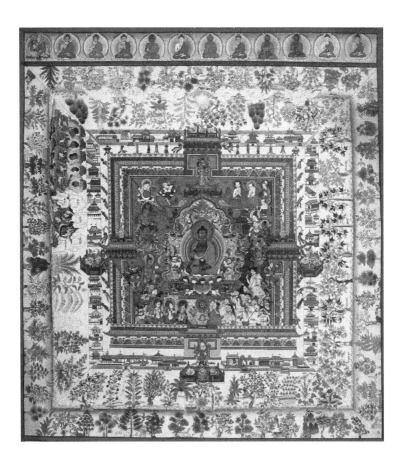

FIG. 2. Medicine Buddha Mandala

Root Tantra, the first of the four volumes. Yuthok first takes us to the central part of the garden, where there is a palace built with the five precious substances and encrusted with various kinds of precious stones. These precious jewels have the power to cure 404 diseases arising from the disorders of the three humors (three principal energies present in the body). They serve to pacify the disturbances of heat and cold and the 1,080 barriers that interfere with good health, and meet all needs and desires. The gems bathe us in light that penetrates us with white, yellow, red, blue, and green, dissolving and inactivating any poisons, spirits, obscurations, presumptions, and fevers. The gems purify us and satisfy our cravings.

Medicine Buddha Mandala

On the walls of the palace are also the gems of the Devas.[3] In addition to the above-mentioned qualities, they also have the ability to protect and to provide clarity, have absolute purity, and provide the ability to speak.

We find also the gems of the bodhisattvas, which have the additional ability to allow us to see the death and rebirth of sentient beings—to realize who is about to become enlightened. Therefore, the Medicine Buddha teaches differently and adequately according to the attitudes and abilities of the disciples.

From the center of Tanadug, we move to the southern garden. Here is the Thunderbolt or "Penetrative" Mountain (Tib. *'bigs byed*, Skt. *Vindhya*), which has the strength and power of the sun. On its slopes grow plants such as pomegranate, black pepper, and long pepper. We find precious metals and all medicinal substances that heal the disorders of the cold. It is a forest full of substances that possess the qualities of heat and sharpness and are hot, sour, and salty in taste. Therapeutic preparations are made from the roots, trunks, branches, leaves, flowers, and fruits, and are fragrant and pleasant. No cold disorder can arise when one can smell their bouquet.

In the northern part of Tanadug is "Snow-Capped" Mountain (Tib. *gangs can*, Skt. *Himavata*), which is imbued with lunar qualities. There

---

[3] Deva (male) or Devi (female) ("those that emanate light"; from the Sanskrit root meaning to shine, emit light) is the Sanskrit word for god, divinity, but also indicates in general a celestial being, demigod, angel.

we find sandalwood trees, camphor, agarwood, and all the remedies that cure the disorders of heat and fever. They taste bitter, sweet, and astringent. They have cooling, soft, and gentle properties. The substances are obtained from any part of the plant from the root to the fruit, and their invigorating fragrances prevent all hot disorders like fever, infections, and inflammations from arising.

The Scheme of Tanadug–Medicine Buddha Mandala

Moving to the east, we find "Fragrant" Mountain (Tib. *spos ngad ldan*). Here grows a forest of arura trees. The arura can cure many types of disor-

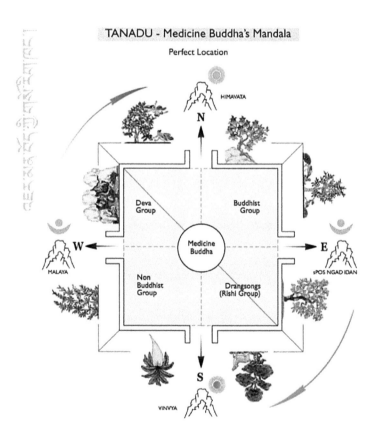

FIG. 3. Medicine Buddha's Mandala

ders. Its roots heal bone pathologies; the trunk cures diseases of the body; the branches heal diseases of channels and ligaments; the bark heals skin disorders; the leaves cure the diseases of the hollow organs, namely, stomach, small intestine, colon, urinary bladder, and gall bladder; the flowers cure diseases of the sense organs; and finally, the fruits cure diseases of the heart and other vital organs.

The five types of arura fruit are endowed with the six tastes, the eight natural powers, the three postdigestive tastes, and seventeen secondary qualities. These fruits heal all types of disorders, and if the scent of these attractive fruits is present, the 404 types of diseases will not manifest.

Visiting the west, we find the "Garlanded" Mountain (Tib. *ma la ya*), where the six excellent medicines grow. They are also known as the Six Good Substances: nutmeg, clove, saffron, bamboo pith, black cardamom, and green cardamom. All diseases are pacified by the five types of calcites, five varieties of mineral exudates, five kinds of medicinal water, and five types of hot springs on these shores.

Around the city, we see fields of saffron and notice the smell of incense. Everywhere abound rocks and salts with individual medicinal properties. Peacocks, cranes, parrots, and other birds sing softly from the treetops. All kinds of animals such as elephants, bears, and musk deer roam the land, and each3 provides excellent remedies.

Returning to the palace, in the central area, on a throne of aquamarine jewels, sits the Master of Medicine, King of Aquamarine Light, the Transcendent Conqueror fully endowed, the Medicine Buddha who is the Master and Guide.

The throne is surrounded by four groups: gods, sages, non-Buddhists, and Buddhists.

Through the divine abilities of the Medicine Buddha, all present are able to understand the instructions received, as if they belonged to the same tradition.

This teaching is called the "Tradition of the Elders." It is just, true, and eliminates the shortcomings of others caused by the three mental poisons of desire, anger, and ignorance. It leaves everyone without defects in body, speech, and mind.

In our journey, we lose the components of space and time as we enter the mandala and become part of one of the four groups mentioned above. There is room for everyone, and all are welcome.

At this point, the Master Medicine Buddha, surrounded by the four groups of disciples, enters into meditative balance and becomes the Sovereign Healer who overwhelms all 404 types of diseases.

From his heart a variety of brightly colored rays are issued in the ten directions, dispelling the mental distortions of all sentient beings and pacifying any distress arising from the three poisons of ignorance.

The light beams return to the heart of the Buddha. From his heart an emanation of the Buddha called Sage Rigpe Yeshe (*Drangsong Rigpai Yeshe*) or Sage of Primordial Wisdom emerges. This manifests in the space in front of the Master, stating introductory words addressed to the group of wise men:

Oh friends, those who just want to be free from anxiety, those who hope to cure diseases; you must learn the quintessential teachings of the science of healing. Whoever wishes to receive the teachings of the Dharma, prosperity, and happiness must learn these quintessential teachings of the science of healing. Whoever wants to liberate all beings from the misery of affliction and aspires to earn the respect of all beings should learn the quintessential teachings of the science of healing.

After he has pronounced these words, from the tongue of the Supreme Master bloom thousands of polychromatic rays of light, which permeate in the ten directions, removing the verbal contamination of all sentient beings and subjugating all the torments and spirits. Subsequently, the light rays are absorbed by the tongue, which expresses the emanation of the words of the Buddha in the form of Sage Yeley Kye (*Drangsong Yid le kye*), that is, the Scholar Who Is Born of the Mind. The Sage performs prostrations and circumambulates the Master, and addresses a question to him on behalf of the assembly of scholars/students:

"O Master, Sage Rigpe Yeshe, how can we acquire generosity toward ourselves and toward others, as we learn the quintessential teachings of the science of healing?"

The Supreme Master replies: "Great Sages, learn the quintessential tradition of the tantra science of healing. Study the eight limbs, learn the eleven principles, learn the fifteen divisions, assimilate the four collections, and study the 156 chapters."

So the Sage Yeley Kye asks: "O Master, how can we understand the quintessential tradition of the tantra science of healing?"

The Master replies: "Oh Great Scholar, listen and study the Four Tantras, which are Root Tantra, Explanatory Tantra, Oral Instruction Tantra, and Final Tantra."

"What are the eight branches that we need to know?" Yeley Kye questions further.

"They are physical disorders, illnesses in children, illnesses in women, diseases caused by spirits, the wounds caused by firearms, poisonings and geriatric disorders including remedies for impotence, infertility and sterility."

Yeley Kye asks again: "What are the eleven principles to learn?"

"They are:

1. The fundamental principles
2. The formation of the body
3. The law of increase and decrease of the disease
4. Behavioral regimens
5. Dietary regimens
6. The principle of pharmacology
7. The use of surgical instruments
8. The principle of maintaining health
9. The concept of diagnosis
10. Methods of healing; and finally
11. The principal functions of the doctor."

"What are the fifteen subdivisions to know?"
The Master replies: "They are:

1. The category of healing disorders of the three humors
2. The treatment of internal disorders
3. The treatment of fevers
4. The treatment of diseases of the upper body
5. The section on healing of vital and hollow organs
6. The treatment of disorders of the genitals
7. The series with respect to therapy in cases of mixed disorders
8. The class that treats complications that arise as result of treatment
9. The therapies used in healing childhood diseases
10. The therapies used in healing gynecological disorders
11. The area that deals with the diseases caused by spirits
12. The healing of wounds caused by weapons

13. The treatment of poisoning

14. The subdivision that encompasses the extraction of the vital essences (rejuvenation, etc.); and finally

15. The category dealing with the increase in fertility."

"What are the four collections to learn?"
"They are:

1. The list on the analysis of the pulse and the examination of urine
2. The list of substances that fight diseases
3. The list of substances that induce evacuations; and
4. The collection of soothing therapies and drastic therapies."

It was also asked of the Master: "Which are the 156 chapters to study?" The Buddha listed the chapters that made up the body of the *Four Tantras* as follows:

1. *The Root Tantra*, with six chapters, is an introduction that sets out the arguments for the foundations of physiology, diagnosis, and treatment methods and provides a list of metaphors used in Sowa Rigpa.

2. *The Explanatory Tantra*, with thirty-one chapters explaining the eleven principles.

3. *The Oral Instruction Tantra*, composed of ninety-two chapters, in which are analyzed the fifteen divisions.

4. *The Final Tantra*, formed by two chapters on diagnosis, ten about medications that calm, seven about substances that promote clearance, and six chapters thaat speak of external therapies, for a total of twenty-five chapters.

These 154 chapters, plus a concluding chapter and another chapter that addresses what kind of student can receive teachings, make a total of 156 chapters.

TABLE 2.1
The Four Tantras

Root Tantra	Explanatory Tantra	Oral Instruction Tantra	Final Tantra
9 branches	11 principles	15 subdivisions	4 collections
6 chapters	31 chapters	92 chapters	25 chapters
			+2 concluding chapters

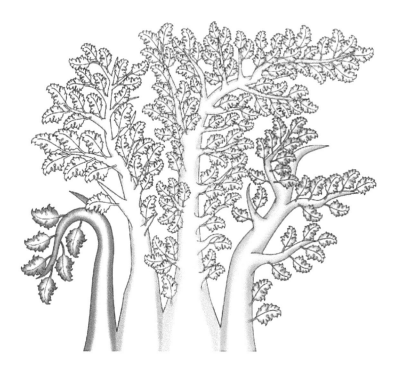

FIG. 4. The Tree of Four Tantras

The goal of the "Four Tantras" is the pursuit of good health, determined by balance on physical, energy, and mental levels.

The Root Tantra (Tsa Gyu) introduces traditional Tibetan medicine. Sowa Rigpa is represented by three trees, also known as The Three Roots:

- The tree of general condition, the tree of physiology and pathology is divided into two trunks: balance (health) and imbalance (disease)
- The tree of diagnosis, divided into three trunks, one for each method of diagnosis: observation, palpation, medical interview or anamnesis
- The tree of therapy, divided into four trunks: diet, lifestyle, medications, and external therapies.

The Explanatory Tantra (She Gyu) addresses the following issues: embryology, anatomy, subtle anatomy (or anatomy of the Vajra Body), physiology, lifestyle, diet, the foundations of pharmacopeia, regular health and prevention, diagnosis, treatment, the ethical code, and the different behaviors of a physician, as well as the use of the instruments in external therapies.

The Oral Instruction Tantra (Man Ngak Gyu) is the largest of the four volumes. It consists of ninety-two chapters, in which are explained pathologies divided by subject: the three humors, internal disorders, fever, upper body, solid organs and hollow organs, disorders and diseases of the genitals, common infections, skin diseases, pediatrics, gynecological disorders, injuries caused by spirits, injuries, poisonings, and recommendations on methods of longevity and ways to increase sexual energy.

The *Final Tantra* or *Tantra of Final Action* (Chima Gyu) examines the practices of a physician and covers:

1. Diagnosis: by examination of the urine and pulse reading
2. Use of pharmacological compounds: decoctions, powders, pills, creams and ointments, medicines made from herbs or ashes, etc.
3. Five actions: diuretics, purges, emetic drugs, inhalation drugs, strong and mild enemas with the aim of obtaining evacuation
4. Six external therapies: bloodletting, moxibustion, compresses, bath therapy, Tibetan massage (*Kunye*), and acupuncture.

Thus ends our introductory journey through the garden of Tanadug and the enumeration of the Four Tantras.

The two main aims for the study of Sowa Rigpa can be summarized as prevention and cure: prevention of diseases by maintaining balance through the use of adequate diet and appropriate lifestyle, and cure of diseases through treatments used to recover a good balance. But what is balance and how does one achieve it? The next chapter will explore the philosophy of Sowa Rigpa to understand how we are created through the five elements of space, wind, fire, water, and earth. This knowledge of the five elements and the derivative concept of three humors, the three energetic principles in our body, is the base of balance.

3

The Philosophy of Sowa Rigpa

THE MAIN PHILOSOPHY of Sowa Rigpa is *tendrel* (*rten 'brel*), the Tibetan word for interdependence or interconnection. It is the concept that nothing can exist by itself, separate from the rest of the universe. All things exist in dependence on one another. *Tendrel* can be compared to a web containing all phenomena that are linked and interconnected based on the theory of cause and effect.

In Sowa Rigpa the five elements and the way they define the nature of mind, body, and environment are fundamental to the practice of medicine and Buddhist tantras.[1]

The Five Elements

In Tibetan, the five elements are called *jungva*. *Va* means elements and *jung* means origin of life, energy, physical body, and mind. Through the omni-

---

[1] *Tantra* refers to a lineage of teaching or system of transmission of a tradition's teachings. Spiritual teachings are passed down orally from master to disciple in a proper and unbroken lineage to ensure their purity and originality.

TABLE 3.1
The Five Elements and Their Properties

ELEMENT	TIBETAN NAME	SOUND	COLOR	SHAPE	GRAPHICAL REPRESENTATION
Space	*Namkha*	*E*	Blue	Oval	
Wind	*Loong*	*Yam*	Green	Semicircle	
Fire	*Me*	*Ram*	Red	Triangle	
Water	*Chu*	*Kham*[2]	White	Circle	
Earth	*Sa*	*Lam*	Yellow	Square	

present elements, everything existing is interconnected and interdependent. The elements are present in our body as well as in our environment, our planet, and our universe. They are space, wind, fire, water, and earth.

Space, the mother of all elements, is immaterial—emptiness. In the absence of space, nothing can exist. The space element is the basis for all the other elements; space contains and surrounds them, and without it nothing can manifest. Space is present in both the internal universe (body and mind) and the external universe (macrocosm).

Wind represents movement. It is the manifestation of growth and development. Wind develops our breath and the skin and is found in the sense of touch.

Fire represents heat. It manifests as maturation. Just as fruit matures through the heat of summer, the body needs fire in order to mature. The heat of fire can be seen in the complexion, the eyes, and the vision.

---

[2] In some five elements purification practices, the sound of the water element can be *Bam*.

Water represents the principle of fluidity, cohesion, and connection. Just as flour needs water to form into sticky dough, the body needs water to bring it into a cohesive whole. It is in the blood, in the lymphatic system, and at the base of the tongue. Further, just as a drop of water entering into the ocean becomes the ocean, water provides the connection and cohesion allowing us to become more than just our singular being.

Earth represents solidity. In our bodies, it is the bones and tendons and provides structure. Earth is the coarsest of elements and is the structure of the world in which we live.

The five elements are interdependent on one another in the same way that all phenomena are interdependent. Their very essence can manifest on subtle levels such as mind, emotions, and energy as well as on the physical level as body or environment.

Subtle and Gross Elements

We recognize the five elements in all manifestations in our life, not only on the gross level (*ragpa*) but also in a more subtle and pure aspect (*tra-wa*). Physical elements originate from elements in a subtle dimension. There, elements are in their pure state, while elements in the physical dimension are in their impure state. In the physical dimension, *jungva*, the five origins or five elements, are manifested as space, wind, fire, earth, and water. As elements of our body they are called the five internal elements (*nang jung*).

The Elements and Their Cycles

As explained in the Buddhist mandala system, we can say that the world consisting of elements is in a constant process of creation and destruction, everything and every being interdependent and interconnected. A mandala shows how everything is created from the five elements.

The five elements are involved in three processes or cycles: creation (birth), maintenance (i.e., living), and destruction (death). In Tibetan, the three processes are called *kye, ne,* and *jig.* They are the most important stages of our life: we are born, we live, and one day we will die.

THE CREATION CYCLE

We are created from the five elements. The creation cycle is a gradual transformation from the space element to the earth element, from emptiness/subtle to form/gross.

SPACE → WIND → FIRE → **WATER** → EARTH

From space, life begins with movement and energy, or breath, which is represented by the wind element. In space manifests wind (motion and energy), without which there would be no life. The movement is a quality of the wind (air). This produces friction and therefore heat and light (fire element). Fire and wind give fluidity to water vapor and clouds and produce rain (water element). The interaction between the wind and fire evaporates the water, and what remains becomes the element of earth (solidity).

THE MAINTENANCE CYCLE

CHILDHOOD → ADULTHOOD → OLD AGE

Since we live by the existence of the five elements as they are all around and within us, we need adequate space, clean air, adequate light, and enough water. We also need healthy food to nurture our earth element. We have this body composed of five elements and we continuously take them in from outside by eating, drinking, breathing, and being. Maintaining the body is a question of balance and the main aim of Sowa Rigpa.

THE DISSOLUTION CYCLE

The body is formed from the elements and when death comes, it destroys itself by dissolving into the elements that constituted it. This cycle goes in the opposite direction, from the earth element back to the space element.

EARTH → **WATER** → FIRE → WIND → SPACE

It begins when the earth element dissolves in water and does not offer more support for awareness. We can observe this stage when we feel as if we are sinking, being crushed by a large weight, or falling into the earth.

People at this stage often ask someone to hold their hand to reduce this feeling and help them better tolerate it. When this perception is over, it means the earth element is completely dissolved in water, so the dying person feels lighter.

Subsequently, water dissolves in fire. During this stage, the body cools slowly, starting from the extremities and moving to the core. Often the person may leak from the orifices: the nose may start to drip, the mouth may drool, the eyes may produce discharge and tears, or the person may become incontinent.

Later, the fire element dissolves in the wind element, causing the loss of internal heat and the body becoming totally cold.

Finally, there is the exhalation of the last breath of air when wind dissolves in space. In this state, the dying person has the sensation of floating on air, the complete opposite of the experience at the beginning.

When wind dissolves, there is no more motion energy or mental energy. At this point, the person is clinically dead and enters into another dimension called bardo, an intermediate state between death and the next life, where physical reality no longer exists.

In the Buddhist tradition, this path is explained with the construction of sand mandalas that use five colors to represent the five elements in the creation cycle (birth); completion of the mandala (life); and finally, its destruction to symbolize impermanence and the dissolution cycle (death). In the end, the sand is thrown away, so that everything dissolves into space! A mandala is not a mere artistic expression; it is something much greater—a teaching of life.

The Five Internal Elements

The elements all have specific features found in all phenomena as well as in our body. Elements in the body are therefore called internal elements. At an embryonic level, each element is involved in the formation of a solid organ,[3] a hollow organ,[4] and major arteries. And each element

---

[3] Five solid organs: heart, lungs, liver, kidneys, spleen.

[4] Six hollow organs: small intestine, large intestine, gall bladder, urinary bladder, genitals, stomach.

itself can be divided into different parts or aspects, e.g., pure/subtle and impure/gross, or different functions. It is considered that the pure part of the element is mainly the corresponding solid organ, but in general all elements in their complex combinations contribute to form the body in its parts and its entirety.

Let's look more specifically at the elements and the corresponding body parts.

Space: In the womb, the pure part of this element creates the heart (solid organ), then a portion of the small intestine (hollow organ); another part, in turn, forms the head.

The space-heart energy is tied to our feelings and emotions that are as empty as infinite space, but also as unlimited. The characteristic emptiness of space can be associated with the heart since the energy of space creates the heart. If we open our heart, it can be endlessly empty and filled with everything, just like space. Our feelings can be endless like space. The emotions influence the heart and head, but also the small intestine, which Sowa Rigpa considers the seat of our emotions. Furthermore, space is found throughout the body in the spaces between the organs, tissues, cells, blood vessels, and lymphatic vessels, etc.

Wind: The pure part creates the lungs (solid organ), then forms the large intestine (hollow organ) and the right leg.

It is the element that supports the lungs, which allow contact between and exchange of the external and internal environment. In addition, a part of us is constituted by air and lives through it. The lungs are connected to the large intestine, so if there is disease in the lungs, there are repercussions at the intestinal level. We find the wind energy in everything that has movement within our body: breathing, heartbeat, intestinal peristalsis, muscle movements, and the continual cell metabolism. Thus, the wind enables the maintenance of psychophysical balance.

Fire: The pure part forms the liver (solid organ) and the impure part forms the gall bladder (hollow organ), then the right arm.

The liver regulates the body temperature with the support of the fire energy. It is the organ that assimilates and filters food, both solid and liquid, and breaks down toxic substances. Fire is also associated with all hepatic tissues.

Water: The pure part forms the kidneys (solid organ) and the impure part forms the urinary bladder (hollow organ), the genitals, and then the left leg.

TABLE 3.2

Physiological Relationships Among Elements, Organs, Functions,
and Parts of the Body

FIVE ELEMENTS	SOLID ORGANS	HOLLOW ORGANS	SENSE ORGANS	SECONDARY FUNCTIONS	SENSES	PARTS OF THE BODY
Space	Heart	Small intestine	Tongue	Control orifices	Hearing (ears)	Forehead
Wind	Lungs	Large intestine	Nose	Breathing	Touch (skin)	Right leg
Fire	Liver	Gall Bladder	Eyes	Temperature; complexion	Vision (eyes)	Right arm
Water	Kidneys	Bladder	Ears	Blood; lymph	Taste (tongue)	Left leg
Earth	Spleen	Stomach	Lips	Muscles, tissues; bones	Smell (nose)	Left arm

The water element is everywhere in the body, since we are mainly composed of liquid, for example, interstitial fluid, lymph fluid, blood, and glandular secretions.

Earth: The pure part forms the spleen (solid organ) and the impure part forms the stomach (hollow organ), then the left arm. The energy of the earth supports the spleen and stomach and produces stability, balance, and strength in the body. We find it in all support components, such as tendons, bones, and tissues.

The Five External Elements

In the physical dimension, *jungva,* the five origins or five elements of space, wind, fire, earth, and water, creates us. At an even grosser dimension they can manifest as five external elements, also called *kham nga* or five astrological elements. The Tibetan word *kham* means energies or external elements (*chi jung*). The five external elements, wood, fire, metal,

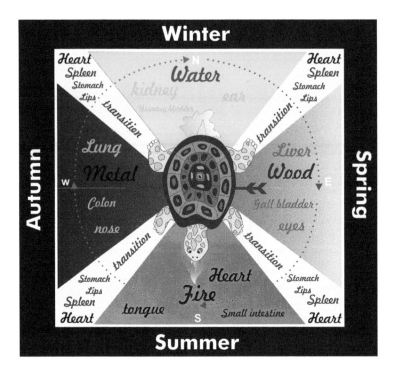

FIG. 5. The Turtle and five external elements

In Tibetan culture, medicine is closely tied to astrological practices. The study of Tibetan astrology starts with a legend about the world's genesis. In the beginning, the universe was a big terrestrial turtle. The turtle's torso was the sky and its flat belly the earth. While hovering in space singing, the Wisdom Buddha shot an arrow of wisdom toward the turtle. The arrow was filled with wood energy and the head with metal. When the arrow hit, the turtle stopped marching. Not recognizing the gift of wisdom, the turtle became angry. It spat fire and urinated on everything. These energies became the seasons, corresponding with the directions, with spring (east) having wood energy, summer (south) having fire energy, autumn (west) having metal energy, and winter (north) having water energy. The intermediate seasons (center) are earth energy. The turtle represents the energy of the universe but also reflects the energy of the individual. It represents both the macrocosm and the microcosm, each influencing the other.

TABLE 3.3
Internal and external energies

External elements	Wood	Fire	Earth	Metal	Water
Internal elements	Space	Fire	Earth	Wind	Water

water, and earth, regulate and maintain the cycle of the seasons. The seasons and environment have an impact on our bodies and influence our organism, and each body part is affected differently.

The most obvious astrological influences affecting health, for both practitioner and patient, are the changes of the seasons. The external elements in the environment are linked to the most salient aspect of energy (that is, the three humors, and how the subtle and gross elements are intricately linked) and are considered influential, particularly on the patient's pulse. There is a method for detecting the pulse that follows a seasonal pattern. In turn, the external elements are related to the five internal elements.

In summary, there are five internal elements, called *jungva nga*, and five external elements, called *kham nga*. The latter should be understood as nature's interactions with the body.

The external elements are important natural forces. If we keep in balance with them, they will have beneficial effects; being out of balance gives rise to disease. Thus, it is important to know the external elements and understand their actions during the different periods of the year, with the purpose of taking care of ourselves and the health of others.

The Seasons

Each season, for the purpose of Sowa Rigpa, lasts three months. Specifically, they consist of ninety days, with seventy-two days of the actual season and eighteen days of transitional period. Table 3.4 shows how our bodies relate to the seasons and the external influences from them.

TABLE 3.4
The internal and external influences of the organs of the human body

INTERNAL	EXTERNAL
Liver—gall bladder	Spring, 72 days
Spleen—stomach	Transition season, 18 days
Heart—small intestine	Summer, 72 days
Spleen—stomach	Transition season, 18 days
Lungs—large intestine	Autumn, 72 days
Spleen—stomach	Transition season, 18 days
Kidneys—urinary bladder	Winter, 72 days
Spleen—stomach	Transition season, 18 days

Spring: March 21 to June 1[5]

During this period, wood energy creates an energy field that, when it reaches the moment of greatest intensity, can influence our organs, particularly the liver. This is due to the stress of the liver working hard during the cold of winter to keep the body warm.

This energy field not only affects the liver, but due to the function of the liver, also can be felt throughout the rest of the body. Therefore, we must be attentive to what we eat and what we do. When the liver is sensitive, we should not drink alcohol. Alcohol increases the strain on the liver's function of detoxification and would further disturb its balance. It is important to remember that allergies also have a hepatic origin.

The wood energy comes from the earth. After seventy-two days this force returns to earth and begins a season of transition.

Transition Season: June 2 to June 20

The energy of the earth affects the spleen and stomach. When the stomach is sensitive, one should eat sparingly.

---

[5] For simplicity, static Western dates are presented. The actual dates vary every year. Those presented are close to correct; for greater accuracy, consult an astrological calendar that gives each of the dates.

Summer: June 21 to September 2

When it is hot, from the earth comes the external element of fire, which influences the heart and small intestine for seventy-two days. Summer is a good season for holidays, but people with sensitive hearts or small intestines have to be careful not to get overheated or too emotionally excited. Because of the fire element, this season is especially dangerous for the elderly if they have heart issues.

Transition Season: September 3 to September 20

The heat is absorbed by the earth for eighteen days. One must again be cautious with the spleen and stomach.

Autumn: September 21 to December 2

In autumn, we have the external element of metal. During the transition period, the late summer heat is reabsorbed by the earth, forming an energy field that emphasizes the many minerals and metals that are present. This season, the lungs and large intestine are sensitive and when out of balance can lead to episodes of coughing, hoarseness, and other airway diseases.

Transition Season: December 3 to December 20

Once again, the energy enters in the intersection to become earth energy.

Winter: December 21 to March 3/4

The cold water coming from either the sky or the earth has an energy field that influences the susceptibility of the urinary bladder and kidneys. One often sees back problems and an increase of urinary frequency and diabetes during this season.

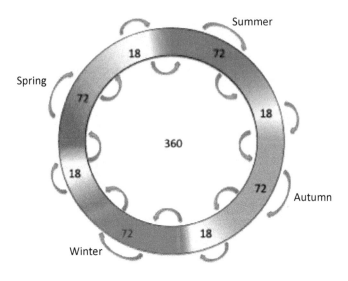

FIG. 6. The cycle of the five external elements according to the seasons

Transition Season: March 4/5 to March 20/21

Eating too quickly, eating while standing up, and eating a bad breakfast are always unhealthy, but during this transitional period when the stomach is most sensitive, they are particularly detrimental. In Sowa Rigpa, digestion is considered as delicate as a child in need of healing. It is the process that allows us to absorb and assimilate the external energy. So it is easy to understand that if digestion is not working properly, it becomes the source of all the imbalances of the body. This can even affect the immune system.

The *Four Tantras* states that we should eat by dividing the stomach into four parts: when eating a meal, two of the four parts should contain food, one part should contain liquid, and one part must be left free to allow for proper digestive function.

In Buddhism, there is a traditional saying: "The Buddha is in our hands; therefore, they are sacred." In the same way, if we follow simple directions, including a good diet and a proper lifestyle, we can achieve and maintain good health! If we fail to maintain a constant adequate diet, at the very least, we must remember to pay greater attention to what we eat during the transition seasons.

Both the external energies and internal elements affect our organs; let's have a closer look now.

The Organs

Heart

The space element is linked to the heart and mind. The fire element also influences the heart. Internal influences like strong emotions, deep feelings, and sorrows also may affect the heart. In the summer, when the external influence of fire energy dominates, these internal influences will be augmented by the external influences, and one is more likely to be susceptible to heart disease and mental problems.

Liver

The liver, in turn, is sensitive to the element fire and the wood energy. The liver is like a laboratory that produces intense heat. It is thus the organ that not only regulates body temperature but also suffers the most when the person is stressed.

In spring, when the wood energy is in full swing, if we indulge in heavy foods rich in fat or drink too much alcohol (external factors), we will become more easily stressed and angry (internal influences). In this case there is a greater chance of getting liver disease.

Kidneys

The kidneys are affected by water, both internally and externally. Therefore, diseases of the urinary tract as well as degenerative joint diseases, also having a cold nature (internal influences), will get worse in winter, especially if we consume foods and drinks that have a cold nature (external influences), such as raw vegetables, barley, or wheat flour.

Lungs

The lungs and large intestine are sensitive to the wind element and the energy of metal. So in autumn, smokers and those who do not wear proper clothing (external factors) may incur cool diseases such as coughing, hoarseness, or colds.

Spleen

The stomach and spleen are influenced by earth. Thus, if during the eighteen days of any period of transition we are immoderate when consuming heavy foods, we will create a general state of fatigue, which can lead to true spleen and gastric diseases.

Connections Between the Organs and Body Parts Through the Five External Elements

Sowa Rigpa includes knowledge about *khams* or the external elements for analyzing the patient's condition. For example, our pulses vary slightly due to changes in the external environment that directly influence our

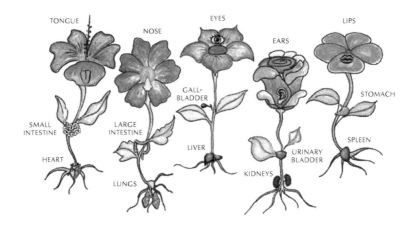

FIG. 7. Interconnectedness of solid organs, hollow organs, and the sense organs

TABLE 3.5
The influences of the seasons/five external elements
on different organs

FIVE EXTERNAL ELEMENTS	SEASON	FLOWER ORGAN	STEM ORGAN	ROOT ORGAN
Wood	Spring	Eyes	Gall bladder	Liver
Fire	Summer	Tongue	Small intestine	Heart
Metal	Autumn	Nose	Large intestine	Lungs
Water	Winter	Kidneys	Urinary bladder	Kidneys
Earth	Transition	Lips	Stomach	Spleen

body. As explained above, each body part is affected differently by the seasons. Therefore, knowledge of the five external elements comes into use with the pulse diagnosis.

There is a direct relationship between organs and body parts, and we can represent them as parts of a flower: the solid organ is the root or seed, the hollow organ is represented by the stem, and the sense organs are the flower, the part that is manifested. When evaluating a patient, using the schematic representation of the flower, we can infer the conditions of internal organs. Figure 7 shows the physiological relationships among elements, seasons, and organs as parts of flowers.

Simplification of the Five Elements

Since the space element penetrates all other elements, when one speaks of four elements, space is implied and understood as the essential element from which the others come. The four elements form the three humors,[6]

---

[6]The three humors: *loong* (Tib. *rLung*), *tripa* (Tib. *mKhrispa*), and *beken* (Tib. *badkan*), known as *nyes pa* in Tibetan, do not have exact corresponding words in English. However, for simplicity and easy understanding, we will refer the humors/*nyes pa* of *loong, tripa*, and *beken as* wind, bile, and phlegm respectively.

The Philosophy of Sowa Rigpa

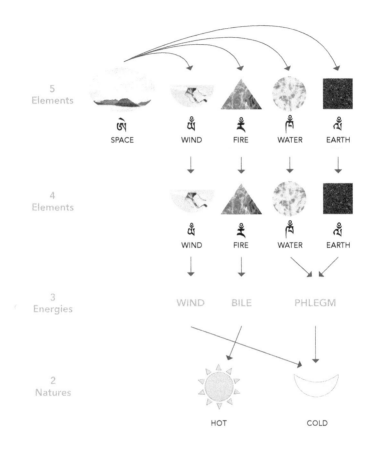

FIG. 8. The five elements and their simplification

the three energies in our body. The element of wind creates the wind humor (Tib. *rLung*). The element of fire creates the bile humor (Tib. *mKhrispa*). Water and earth create the phlegm humor (Tib. *badkan*).

Considering the characteristics of humors, we can construct an equilateral triangle, knowing that at the apex, the neutral element of the wind can have two opposite effects, supporting and increasing the heat energy (*tsawa*) or the cold energy (*drangwa*). These are known as the two natures of diseases. Therefore, we have neutral: wind; hot: bile; cold: phlegm.

The neutral energy of the wind can move to one of the two extremes of hot and cold. The *Four Tantras* explain that the energy from the sun

Wind / Loong

Bile / Tripa

Phlegm / Beken

FIG. 9. Graphic representation of three humors

is hot and the energy from the moon is cold, so if the wind joins one of these two, it gives it support. This is also observed in nature. For example, if there is wind in the winter, you will feel cold, but if you blow on a fire, it ignites with more energy and the wind becomes hot.

Despite the wind humor having a neutral characteristic, it is considered an element of cold nature. The pathologies related to wind will also be cold in nature.

In brief:

five elements: space, wind, fire, water, and earth
four elements: wind, fire, water, and earth
three humors: wind, bile, and phlegm
two natures of diseases: hot and cold

Based on the combination of the three humors, each of us is assigned a constitutional type or typology. The ratio of wind, bile, and phlegm leads to different physical and psychological characteristics. As long as the humors exist in the personal predestined proportions, body and mind are in a state of balance. If the balance of one or more humors is disturbed, it can be considered the basis of disease. We have to keep this concept in mind at all times in order to maintain a healthy balance of body, energy, and mind.

Once we are able to detect the state of the five elements or three humors that may be in excess, deficiency, or disorder in a person, we will be able to use the most appropriate treatment to rebalance the energy through diet, lifestyle, external therapies, and/or medicines.

The Three Humors

The three humors are the foundation of Sowa Rigpa, derived from the five elements. They are wind/*loong*, bile/*tripa*, and phlegm/*beken*.

Creation starts in the womb. First the elements are formed, then the energy centers, followed by the energy channels, organs, and humors. The first element that develops in the fetus is the wind, giving rise to the wind humor (bear in mind that space must be present before all other elements). The second element is fire, from which bile is derived. And finally, the water and earth elements combine and give rise to phlegm.

The wind humor lies in the pelvic area and down the pelvic basin and is related to its support function.

TABLE 3.6
Emotions and corresponding humors

PSYCHOLOGICAL IMBALANCE	HUMORS
Attachment—desire (*dho chags*)	Wind/*loong*
Hatred—aversion (*she dang*)	Bile/*tripa*
Ignorance—delusion (*ti mook*)	Phlegm/*beken*

Bile is located in the trunk, at the center of the chest, and is responsible for the metabolic heat that allows one to digest food.

Phlegm is located from the top of the chest to the crown of the head.

The three humors are called *nyes pa* in Tibetan. This term also means an error or imbalance, because the diseases of body and mind are a result of an imbalance of the three humors.

Wind/Loong

Loong is translated as wind or air, although an older meaning is movement. There are two types of wind/*loong*: subtle wind or *tra loong* (Tib. *phra rLung*) and gross wind or *rag loong* (Tib. *rag rLung*).

In Tibetan culture, the subtle wind is the combination of a dynamic component and a static/stable aspect (consciousness). The dynamic aspect, the vibration of the mind, is in continual movement. Our thoughts are constantly on the move, day and night, through ideas, feelings, memories, and dreams. Movement and awareness are mental aspects that are mixed together in a perfect way; we can imagine them as two sides of the same coin.

It is said that the consciousness is like a person without legs who can see, think, listen, and be aware but cannot move, while the dynamic part

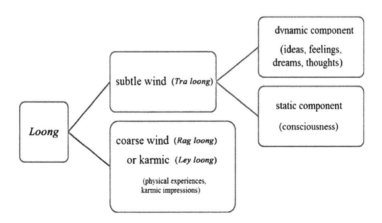

FIG. 10. The Representation of Wind / *Loong* humor.

is like a blind horse that has the power to move, run, and walk but does not know where to go. If the individual without legs is able to mount and guide the blind horse, it will be a perfect situation where the conscious movement can guide one in the right direction. This fusion is a condition called *loong sem* (wind mind).

When one calms down the motion, i.e., the continuous vibration of the mind, the wind is harmonized awareness, resulting in a stabilized mind.[7] This allows one to clearly "see" ultimate reality—the essence of what surrounds us—with an unbiased, nonjudgmental, and nondual attitude. This state, achieved through the practice of meditation, enables us to dissolve the coarse elements in the subtle. This allows our energy to go beyond perceived physical boundaries and puts the mind in a stable contemplative state, omnipresent as space. It is not easy to experience this subtle wind energy (*tra loong*), which is constantly overwhelmed by the gross wind energy (*rag loong*).

When gross wind is predominant, we have no power over our mind, our body, or our emotions. With meditative practice, we can develop the subtle wind energy and then control our mental state. The gross wind can also be called *ley loong* (karmic wind), because it is controlled by the law of karma (cause and effect) and as such, is in continuous motion.

To sum up, the subtle wind operates more on a mental level. Its impure aspect is our normal mind and its processes, while its pure aspect is

---

[7] The meditative techniques can be grouped into two basic types: stabilizing (absorptive) and analytical. In fact, any form of meditative practice can only fall into the category of absorption of the object of meditation or its analysis. Both are methods to cultivate the attention, but their effects are different. Stabilizing meditation (*samatha* or *shi ney* in Tibetan) consists of developing the ability to focus, without interruption, on a subject (e.g., breathing, a concept, an image, a statue) and become familiar with it, abandoning any thought. This does not mean completely emptying the mind. The fruit of this type of meditation is not the absence of thoughts, but the fact that they are no longer harmful when they arise. One is able to let them pass naturally rather than becoming attached to them. The analytical meditation (*vipasyana*) is penetrating and introspective and creates profound insight into the ultimate nature of the subject chosen. Vipasyana consists of intellectual understanding. Topics commonly include the reality of things (characterized by impermanence and selflessness); the law of interdependence (analyzing the law of cause and effect); emptiness (the fact that all phenomena lack an autonomous and intrinsic nature); the benefits of patience; the disadvantages of anger, etc. These two types of meditation are complementary, and to transform the mind, they are often used together in a single meditation session.

TABLE 3.7

Five types of winds / *loong*

WIND	LOCATION	FUNCTIONS
Life-supporting wind / *sog zin loong* (Tib.) *srog dzin rLung*	Head	1. The principal wind, from which derive the other four winds 2. Connects the body with mind and energy 3. Controls functions such as swallowing, breathing, salivation, sneezing, and hiccups 4. Provides clarity to the intellect and to the sensory perceptions and ensures the functioning of memory.
Ascending wind / *gen gyu loong*(Tib. *rGyen rGYu rLung*)	Chest (thorax)	1. Controls speech 2. Generates physical and mental strength 3. Clears the complexion 4. Gives courage 5. Gives the ability to focus, will power, and clear memory.
All-pervasive wind / *khyab je loong* (Tib. *khyab Byed rLung*)	Heart	1. Produces the heartbeat 2. Encourages the movement of the heart and body 3. Responsible for the physical movements of walking 4. Opens and closes the doors of the senses and the skin pores.
Wind that increases metabolic heat / *me nyam loong* (Tib. *me mNyam rLung*)	Stomach, small intestine	1. Presides over digestion and assimilation of food 2. Regenerates body constituents.
Descending wind / *thur sel loong* (Tib. *thur Sel rLung*)	Colon, rectum	1. Regulates the retention and elimination of reproductive fluids (sperm and egg), blood, feces, and urine 2. Assists with delivery during childbirth.

TABLE 3.8

Characteristics of wind/*loong*

CHARACTERISTICS	MANIFESTATIONS
Rough (*zub*)	Mental stress; skin rough, dry
Light (*yang*)	Mind that produces many thoughts; head in the clouds
Cold (*drang*)	Cold feeling that runs through the body, shivering; depression
Subtle (*tra*)	Pain that may be present anywhere in the body; recurrent thoughts, fixations
Hard (*sra*)	Muscle stiffness; stubbornness
Mobile (*yo*)	Easily changeable mind; inability to stand firm

also called our wisdom mind, which is beyond cause and effect. The gross wind, on the other hand, works more on a physical level, and drives our body and its functions.

There are five gross winds, discussed in detail in table 3.7.

Sog means vital energy, while *zin* means support. *Sog zin loong*, the wind that sustains life, sustains the other four winds. It is present within the forehead and brain (in Tibetan the brain is called "ocean nerves") and from there descends to the esophagus.

All winds act directly on physiological functions and thus influence the health of the body. The wind that helps digestion brings into action the muscles of the organs that assimilate food; the descending wind allows the removal of waste products; the ascending wind is related to language. The all-pervasive wind has a more extensive action. On top of the functions mentioned above, it is responsible for our sleeping experiences. As energy rises in the central channel[8] from the abdominal area to the head, dreams appear. That is why dreams are largely made up of experiences that remain stored in the unconscious mind.

When we experience deeper emotions such as passion, which initially we may not even realize, our body shows outward manifestations such as loss of appetite or bowel irregularity, originating from the small in-

---

[8] One of three main energetic channels, through which the energy linked to the Wind humor flows.

testine. Something similar happens when you have digestive problems; the main cause is mental stress, because the major wind is in the mind. Changes in wind energy can result in imbalances in body and mind. If we are imbued with negative emotions, it is very likely reflected in our internal organs. There will be manifestations of psychosomatic illnesses and other problems like constipation, diarrhea, dysmenorrhea, headache, liver disease, etc.

Table 3.8 analyzes some manifestations of wind/*loong* imbalances and how they are related to the characteristics of wind.

TABLE 3.9
Five types of bile/*tripa*

BILE	LOCATION	FUNCTIONS
Digestive bile *juje tripa /* (Tib. *ju Byed mKhrispa*)	Duodenum, small intestine	1. Regulates the digestion of foods and separation of nutrients and non-nutritive substances 2. Increases body heat 3. Strengthens and sustains the other types of bile.
Color-producing bile / *dang gyur tripa* (Tib. *mDangs gyur mKhrispa*)	Liver	1. Produces the various pigmentations of bile and other body constituents 2. Performs the function of red blood cells in Western medicine.
Energizing bile; also called bile of desire, ego / *doob je tripa* (Tib. *sGrub Byed mKhrispa*)	Heart	1. Produces pride, the speed of thought, courage, and sense of dignity 2. Constitutes the basis of ego 3. Confers the ability to concentrate the mind and energy to complete projects.
Vision-producing bile / *thong je tripa* (Tib. *mThong Byed mKhrispa*)	Eyes	1. Determines the visual perception.
Complexion clearing bile / *dok sel tripa* (Tib. *mDog gSal mKhrispa*)	Skin	1. Determines the characteristic color of the-complexion.

Bile/Tripa

Bile humor is hot energy. The word in Tibetan means fire or burn. It is connected to the gall bladder. The subdivisions of bile are listed in table 3.9.

Digestive bile is headquartered in the small intestine and as its name implies, it is associated with digestion, aided by the metabolic wind, which increases the heat. Digestive bile is also associated with the regulation of body temperature and supports the other four types of bile.

Color-producing bile gives coloration; it is linked to the process of skin pigmentation. The color of our skin is not fixed but can be changed if we apply actions to purify it.

The bile of desire, also called bile of ego, is headquartered in the heart. At a mental level it reinforces the sense of self, mental strength, pride, and determination to achieve desired goals, but also reinforces selfishness. One cause of depression is lack of this energy. This bile needs to be in balance, without excesses; then it enables us to trust ourselves. In Buddhist religious practice, one often visualizes oneself as a deity in order to develop divine pride. This leads to a balance of this kind of bile.

The visual bile in the eyes allows us to see colors and shapes clearly. It is also responsible for the intensity of our inner vision, making our dreams feel as real as our waking experience.

The seven characteristics of bile/*tripa* are described in table 3.10. Obviously, the presence of one or more characteristics may indicate an imbalance of this humor.

TABLE 3.10
Characteristics of bile/*tripa*

CHARACTERISTICS	MANIFESTATIONS
Oily (*num*)	Greasy skin, fat that melts in the heat
Acute (*no*)	Acute pain, rapid maturation of the disorders; sharp mind
Hot (*tsa*)	High body temperature; anger, impulsiveness
Light (*yang*)	Rapid response to treatment, but also to the manifestation of the disease; easy irritability and rapid return to calm
Smelly (*dri nam*)	Profuse sweating with strong and pungent odor
Purgative (*tru*)	Excess liquid from the gall bladder that pours into the small intestine and has a purgative effect
Liquid/moist (*sher*)	Excess liquid and dampness causes dysentery

Phlegm/Beken

The term *beken* literally means water and earth. The phlegm humor has a cold and watery nature. Primarily it is found in bodily fluids like blood, lymph, secretions, and excretions, though it is also found in all other parts of the body to a lesser degree since we are mostly composed of water.

When this humor is balanced, it allows one to have a positive mind that is stable, peaceful, and satisfied. In the case of excess or disorder, to rebalance phlegm, it is useful to administer the opposite energy, i.e., heat (e.g., moxa or wraps/compresses).

The phlegm humor also has five subdivisions: satisfying, supporting, connective, mixing, and tasting. Their locations and functions are described in table 3.11.

TABLE 3.11
Five types of phlegm/*beken*

PHLEGM	LOCATION	FUNCTIONS
Supporting phlegm / *ten je beken* (Tib. *rTen Byed Badkan*)	Thorax	1. Supports other types of phlegm-regulating functions 2. Regulates the fluids in the body
Mixing phlegm / *nyak je beken* (Tib. *myag Byed Badkan*)	Stomach	Mixes and breaks down liquid and solid foods into smaller pieces.
Tasting phlegm / *nyong je beken* (Tib. *myong Byed Badkan*)	Tongue	Allows the perception of flavors.
Satisfying phlegm / *tsim je beken* (Tib. *tsim Byed Badkan*)	Head	Determines the joyous feeling of fullness in the experiences of the six senses.[9]
Connective phlegm / *jor che beken* (Tib. *byor Byed Badkan*)	Joints	1. Responsible for ligaments and the lubrication of the bones and all joints 2. Allows for flexibility of movement.

[9] In Buddhist culture there are six senses, organized by the organs that allow us to have sensations: the five sense organs—eyes, ears, nose, tongue, skin, which respectively allow contact with colors, visible forms, sounds, smells, tastes, and tangible objects. From this contact derives five types of physical sensation: visible, sonic, olfactory, gustatory, tactile (e.g., sensations of heat, cold, itching, joint pain); and the body (or faculty) mind that perceives all objects that are not material, that is, the mental sensations such as ideas, thoughts, ideas, dreams, memories, feelings, and emotions such as fear or friendship.

TABLE 3.12

Characteristics of *beken*

CHARACTERISTICS	MANIFESTATIONS
Oily (*num*)	Understood as body fat, overweight
Cold (*sil*)	Cold skin, feeling deep cold
Heavy (*ci*)	Understood as a serious body, imposing
Dull (*tul*)	Physically lazy, slow; mental attitude dull
Smooth (*jam*)	Skin and physical structure smooth; entally indicates kindness
Stable (*ten*)	Mental and physical stability
Viscous (*jar pag*)	Presence of substances like mucus

The satisfying phlegm rebalances disorders from "wind that sustains life" when there is a preponderance of desire, lust, restlessness, or a feeling of dissatisfaction. The supporting phlegm is the root of the other four phlegms. Connective phlegm can be thought of as the glue of the body, providing connection between the disparate parts. The mixing phlegm churns or mixes food and is connected to mechanical digestion. Tasting phlegm gives rise to the six tastes, each of which influences the body in specific ways.

Table 3.12 presents the characteristics of unbalanced phlegm and how they can manifest physically or mentally.

Bile and phlegm both have the characteristic of oiliness. However, "oily" in bile refers to greasy skin, a quality that always manifests on the surface. The oily characteristic in phlegm is understood as a tendency toward increased weight, as body fat. This refers to the inside of the body and causes a decrease in temperature and also slows down the movements. Such excess phlegm is treated by applying heat and exercise. It can be stated that the best cure for phlegmatic people is physical activity!

Wind and phlegm both have the quality of cold, but with wind cold is transient and superficial, manifesting in chills and feeling cold in one's limbs, while with phlegm cold is a profound experience that is felt deeply and is often reported as a feeling of freezing.

The Subtle Anatomy

The subtle anatomy, also called the anatomy of the vajra body, is the study of the human energy system. In Tibetan medicine, the subtle anatomy is originally mentioned by Yuthok the Younger in the *Yuthok Nyingthig*[10] text. Learning the subtle anatomy in connection with medicine will help us gain deeper knowledge and suggest more possible ways to maintain and restore balance. In the body there is a network of 80,000 subtle channels where the wind energy circulates, but for medical purposes we focus on only some parts of it. The main components taken into consideration here are the five chakras and three main energy channels, as well as thirteen internal and six external channels (see chapter 8).

The Five Chakras

The chakras are called in Tibetan *tsa khor*, *tsa* means channel and *khor* means wheel. *Tsa khor* is often translated as "wheels formed by the channels." Occasionally it is also referred to as *khorlo*, which means wheel. *Chakra* is a Sanskrit word that means mandala, although it is commonly used with a wider meaning.

The chakras are in close relationship with the three channels. The center channel is directly in the midline of the body, in front of the spine. Flanking the central channel are the left and right channels. These intersect at several points, forming the so-called "ties of the center channel" (Tib. *tsa dud*). The *tsa dud*, the knots where the channels meet, are each connected to one of the five elements and are the origins of the chakras.

The function of the chakras is partly analogous to the function of the endocrine glands as described by Western medicine. The endocrine glands are mainly responsible for the production and secretion of hormones. These chemical messengers are carried by the blood to various parts of the body and, by action in the nervous system, have the ability to influence our emotions and our energy. Emotions and energy, in turn, also affect the functioning of the endocrine glands and consequently the production of hormones.

---

[10] *Yuthok Nyingthig* means "The Innermost Essence of the Teachings of Yuthok." The *Yuthok Nyingthig* root text was composed in the twelfth century as part of what later came to be known as "The Two Jewels" by Yuthok the Younger. *Gyud Shi*, the *Four Tantras*, is the first "jewel" and the main text of Sowa Rigpa. *Yuthok Nyingthig* is regarded as the second "jewel" and explains Yuthok's spiritual teachings. Yuthok considered spiritual practice to be an integral part of every physician's training. Therefore, *Yuthok Nyingthig* is an important spiritual practice for physicians and practitioners of traditional Tibetan medicine.

However, while the endocrine system regulates the internal response of the organism through production of chemical mediators, the system of chakras and the channels are connected to sounds, colors, and energies, which have a profound effect on the innermost functions of the body.

TABLE 3.13

The chakras

Dechen or head chakra, also called "great bliss" or "great pleasure." Its color is white, its sound is OM, and it has thirty-two petals arranged like an open umbrella. Located inside the head, it corresponds to the spot in the midline between the eyebrows. It is the point where the sexual energy and mind join during sexual union.

Long chod or throat chakra, also called "enjoyment" or "experience." It is red and has sixteen petals, its sound is A, and its shape is similar to a snake coiled in a spiral. It is located in the area of the seventh cervical vertebra. Here the vital energy collects during sleep, causing the mind to produce dreams. It allows the experience of six tastes (sweet, sour, salty, bitter, pungent, and astringent) and influences the vibration of the word.

Cho or heart chakra, also considered "the Dharma of phenomena," understood as the space containing emotions and feelings. It has eight blue petals, its sound is HUM, and its shape resembles a ball. It is located near the sixth thoracic vertebra. Here remain the vital energy and the mind during dreamless sleep. The heart chakra allows the proper functioning of sensory perception and the different qualities corresponding to the levels of consciousness.

Trul pai or navel chakra, also called "manifestation" or "emanation" because it is believed that incarnation has its origins in the navel. It has sixty-four petals arranged radially like spokes on a wheel, its color is orange, its sound is SO, and it is located at approximately the third lumbar vertebra. It is in this center that life force is generated as the location of digestion. This chakra is where the energy and the mind are vital during the waking state.

Dekyong or base chakra or genital chakra, meaning "sustaining the bliss." The head chakra and the base chakra have similar names because the head chakra is where an orgasm first manifests and the base chakra is where it ends. It has thirty-two petals that resemble the foliage of a tree, its color is green, and its sound is HÁ. It is the place of reproductive functions. Together with the head, it is the chakra where the vital energy and the mind join during sexual union.

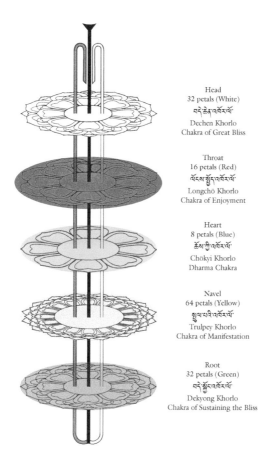

Head
32 petals (White)
བདེ་ཆེན་འཁོར་ལོ་
Dechen Khorlo
Chakra of Great Bliss

Throat
16 petals (Red)
ལོངས་སྤྱོད་འཁོར་ལོ་
Longchö Khorlo
Chakra of Enjoyment

Heart
8 petals (Blue)
ཆོས་ཀྱི་འཁོར་ལོ་
Chökyi Khorlo
Dharma Chakra

Navel
64 petals (Yellow)
སྤྲུལ་པའི་འཁོར་ལོ་
Trulpey Khorlo
Chakra of Manifestation

Root
32 petals (Green)
བདེ་སྐྱོང་འཁོར་ལོ་
Dekyong Khorlo
Chakra of Sustaining the Bliss

The chakras are formed during development of the fetus. In the fifth week of gestation, at the level of the third lumbar vertebra, the navel chakra (*trul pai*) and its four branches like a mandala take form. This development is very crucial for the development of the baby—giving the very essence and energy for the rest of its life.

From the sixth week, from the navel chakra the channels are formed, followed by the base chakra at the genitals and then the heart chakra. In the seventh week the throat chakra forms, and finally the head chakra.

In Sowa Rigpa, there are also four minor chakras in the body: (1) the wind chakra located at the elbows, (2) the water chakra in the knees, (3) the fire chakra found in the palms of the hands, and (4) the blood chakra on the soles of the feet.

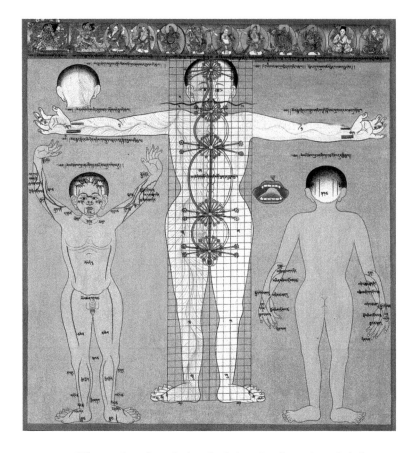

FIG. 11. Tibetan thangka painting depicting the channels and chakras.

The Three Channels

According to Sowa Rigpa, there are also many subtle energy channels, lines of energy, flowing inside our body. The three most important flow in the anterior trunk, in front of the spine. In the right channel flows solar energy (Tib. *roma*), in the left channel flows lunar vitality (Tib. *kyangma*). At the center, anterior to the spine, is the central channel (Tib. *uma*, in between), which is connected to wind/*loong*.

The upper end of the central channel reaches the point called "heavenly gate" or "crown point," located at the top of the head. The apex of each channel is located on its respective nostril. The lower end of the central channel reaches the genitals.

The right half of the body is influenced by the channel *roma* and is related to solar energy, heat, and bile/*tripa*. The liver and gall bladder are located in the right half of the body, and this part is related to the control of body temperature.

The left side of the body, in turn, is influenced by the channel *kyangma* and is related to lunar energy, cold, and phlegm/*beken*.

These three main channels—*roma*, *kyangma*, and *uma*—determine the formation of all other channels and ensure the presence of energy in the other channels and organs of the body.

Solar energy, according to the subtle anatomy, has feminine characteristics, while the moon has masculine characteristics.[11]

The central channel *uma* blows the primordial wisdom wind (*yeshe loong*), which is an indestructible power not influenced by the mind and over which the action wind (karmic wind or *ley loong*) has no power, so it is immune to the law of cause and effect. The central channel is the central mother of perfect balance. It is also called the mother of liberation or realization. Here one experiences the state of nonduality, a pure state of no thoughts.[12]

Beyond the central channel, other channels branch out and become progressively smaller. Within them flow various types of wind energies. Generally, they can be referred to as *ley loong*, that is, karmic winds, which are subject to the law of cause and effect.[13]

---

[11] The Tibetan names of the three main channels all end in *ma*, an ending that indicates the feminine gender. It denotes the three main channels as the "queen" channels, as all other channels are formed from them. These three branch off into estimated 24,000 channels each, totaling 72,000 subtle channels.

[12] One can harness the power of wisdom wind through spiritual practices and thereby rebalance the other gross winds. The spiritual aspect of realization functions mainly through the central channel. The famous Indian Buddhist yogi Saraha said that when our wind energy and our consciousness enter the central channel, all our common or normal perception completely disappears so that our mind is free of the dualism of self and other. This is called the experience of realization.

[13] A fundamental concept in both Tibetan medicine and Buddhism is that no effect exists without a cause. Effects can then become causes, leading to further effects. This ongoing cycle is what constitutes samsara. By understanding the nature of samsara, we can create more balance in our life, for example, by correctly identifying the cause of illness and successfully avoiding it. A healthy state, consisting of the balance of body, energy, and mind, is our only tool within samsara to reach for a state beyond samsara's suffering. So, the path of healing is not only a path of physical and mental balance but also a path to absolute balance.

These karmic winds can be brought into equilibrium through practices such as yoga and breathing exercises. Meditating in the sevenfold meditation posture or vajra position with legs crossed, back straight, and eyes half closed allows us to modify the route of movement of the descending wind (*thur sel loong*, which is a gross or karmic wind, and one of the five divisions of the wind humor discussed above) that is well targeted to the central channel, where it dissolves. This rebalances the energy, which explains why buddhas are often portrayed in the vajra position.

Ancient practitioners such as both the elder and the younger Yuthok Yonten Gonpo sought to go beyond the gross elements and work with the subtle, seeking to develop and to manage them adequately. When one gains control over the elements, the gross part is absorbed into the subtle. Once this happens, there is no imbalance, injury, or illness, and everything is completely at peace. Sowa Rigpa and its related practices not only help one to maintain health but can also help one to develop oneself through the subtle elements as a means to attain enlightenment.[14] Hence, everything comes from the five elements; we are born from them, we live in them, and we die by them. Not only that, we attain enlightenment through the five elements!

Ninefold Purification Breathing

The ninefold purification breathing (Tib. *rlung ro bsal ba*, meaning expelling the dead wind) is a meditative breathing exercise used to balance the three humors, the three energies in the body. Each humor has a corresponding channel and associated emotion, element, color, and representative animal, as shown in table 3.14.

---

[14] According to Yuthok's *Four Tantras* and the *Yuthok Nyingthig*, his heart teachings, there are two aspects of balance: relative and absolute. Sowa Rigpa therefore has two fundamental meanings, "Healing Science" and "Nourishment of Awareness," which reveal the twin aspects of health: the relative balance of mind, body, and energy, governed by the law of cause and effect; and the absolute balance beyond condition or duality. The relative balance builds up a base from which one can work toward the absolute balance.

TABLE 3.14

The three humors, channels, and associated characteristics

	ROMA RIGHT CHANNEL	*UMA* CENTRAL CHANNEL	*KYANGMA* LEFT CHANNEL
Emotion	Anger	Attachment	Ignorance
Element	Fire	Wind	Water and earth
Humor	Bile	Wind	Phlegm
Energy	Solar	Neutral	Lunar
Color	Red	Blue	White
Animal	Snake	Rooster	Pig

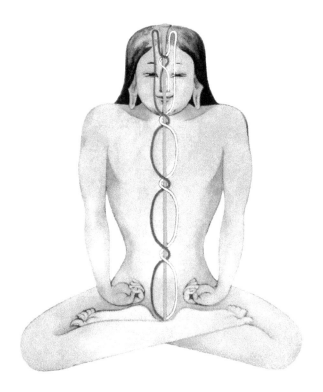

FIG. 12. The sevenfold meditation posture, three channels, and the intersections being the location of the five chakras.

Phase One: Seven Meditation Postures

Start the breathing exercise by sitting in the Sevenfold Meditation Posture of Vairocana (Tib. *rnam snag chos bdun*):

1. Sit cross-legged, ideally in the full lotus position (balances descending wind).
2. Keep the spine straight, like a stack of golden coins (balances fire-accompanying wind).
3. Clasp the hands in vajra fists (thumb pressed on the base of the ring finger) and press on the groins (balances descending wind).
4. Touch the tongue to the palate, just behind the teeth (balances life-sustaining wind).
5. Lift the shoulders up with straightened arms, like folded eagle's wings (balances all-pervading wind).
6. Tuck chin in slightly, like a swan (balances ascending wind).
7. Gaze at the tips of your nose, or into space beyond (balances life-sustaining wind).

Phase Two: Empty Body Visualization

Visualize the form of your body as hollow, empty, a clear shell of luminosity. Within your body are the three channels. Visualize them as empty tubes. The central channel is blue, the right channel is red, and the left channel is white.

The right channel is solar energy, representing the emotion of anger and bile, the fire element. The left channel is lunar, representing ignorance and phlegm, the water and earth element. The central channel is wind energy as well as the emotion of attachment. The impurities of the right, left, and central channels are symbolized by a snake, pig, and rooster respectively. These represent the three fundamental poisons of conditioned existence, the primary root cause of suffering.

Rest in this visualization of the pure dimension of the body, empty body and empty channels, for a moment.

Phase Three: Ninefold Purification Breathing

For all of the following hand positions, the thumb presses on the base of the ring finger, making a partial vajra fist.

1. Exhale completely. Close your left nostril with your left index finger; inhale while bringing the right index finger to the right nostril. Visualize inhaling pure rainbow light through the right nostril, bringing it down the right channel together with your finger. At the navel level, hold your breath and turn your index finger and hand up, leading the energy up the left channel. Exhale through the left nostril, visualizing all impurities of anger as red smoke or little snakes being expelled; release the left index finger from the left nostril while closing the right index finger over the right nostril.

2. Repeat the process for the left channel with reversed hands. All impurities of ignorance are released as whitish-gray smoke or little pigs.

3. Guide with both hands as you inhale with both nostrils to cleanse all channels. Exhale all impurities of attachment as dark smoke or little roosters through both nostrils.

These three breaths are one cycle. Repeat the breathing sequence at least three times to complete the nine breaths.

Phase Four: Mindful Breathing Practice

Sitting in the sevenfold meditation posture, take seven or twenty-one deep breaths. Each deep breath consists of three phases: inhalation, retention, and exhalation. The count for each breath sequence is 4-3-5 (inhaling-holding-exhaling).

You can combine this breathing practice with visualization, inhaling five rainbow colors (blue, green, red, white, yellow), representing the five pure elements of space, wind, fire, water, and earth. While exhaling, radiate light out through the pores of the skin.

Through such mindful breathing practices, we can rebalance our energies. There are three aspects of balance: body, energy, and mind. They are in constant interaction and thus influencing one another. Wind energy and the channels are the connection between body and mind. By working with our energy, we can affect the health of our physical body and our mind.

4

The Three Levels of Balance

As INTRODUCED in chapter 2, *The Root Tantra* (*Tsa Gyu*) explains the three roots of Sowa Rigpa. This metaphor not only stands for the knowledge and works of a physician but also emphasizes the importance of *The Root Tantra*; any plant can only grow if the roots are healthy. In this aspect, *The Root Tantra* is the base of Sowa Rigpa. The first root is referred to as the tree of health and disease. It consists of two trunks, one the balanced state and the other the imbalanced state of the body. The trunk of health/balance has three branches that described the state of energy, body, and mind.

In Sowa Rigpa, health is understood as balance, a dynamic condition found when there is a harmonious relationship of energy, physical body, and mind. When our energies are in balance we feel good; if they start to destabilize, we feel unwell. Energy can destabilize in many ways—there may be a problem with the relationships between them; energy can go the wrong direction or it can stagnate. As energy follows the mind, obsessive thoughts or too many thoughts can create excessive uninterrupted movement, a kind of constant vibration that is dysfunctional.

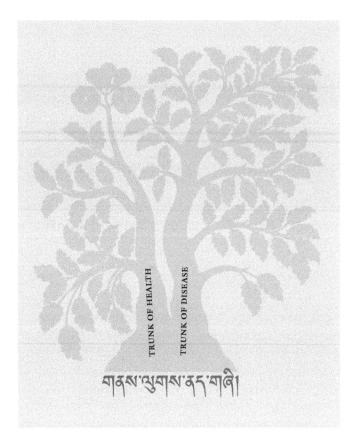

FIG. 13. The Tree of Health and Disease

Balance of Energy

The first branch of the trunk of health represents the three humors. On this branch are five blue leaves, five yellow leaves, and five white leaves, representing the five divisions of each of the humors: wind/*loong*, bile/*tripa*, and phlegm/*beken* respectively. As mentioned in the previous chapters, these are the three energetic principles that allow us to live, to nourish ourselves, to grow, and to relate to the world around us.

Modern physics tells us that everything in the universe is vibrating in constant motion—all of the numberless atoms and subatomic particles, living beings, planets, stars, galaxies. We call this vibration energy. Everything in our bodies is also in constant motion: mind, heartbeat, blood circulation, respiration, intercellular exchange, firing neurons. In the body there are trillions of cells living by virtue of this vibration, performing interdependent functions with the purpose of communication, exchange, and support. Without vibration there is no life, and without life there is no body!

In Tibetan medicine, this vibration, or energy, in our bodies can be hot, cold, or neutral. In the classification system of Sowa Rigpa, wind/*loong* is said to have neutral energy, which has a peculiar characteristic of motion and strength that can influence either bile/*tripa* (heat energy) or phlegm/*beken* (cold energy). Therefore, wind is the most important element and humor.

Bile/*tripa*, as hot energy, is the basis for our body temperature and metabolic heat for digestion and metabolism.

Phlegm/*beken*, as cold energy, constitutes our cells and body fluids, forming the structure of our life.

To understand the physiological functions of the body, we look at the second branch in the trunk of health/balance.

Balance of the Physical Body

The second branch of the trunk of health has seven leaves representing the seven constituents that form the basic foundation of the body. The human body extracts physical substances through the food we ingest. Food is chemically broken down into small parts and then absorbed in the digestive tract. These parts or constituents are then transported to different places in the body for further processing or use. Each has a pure part that forms other constituents and an impure part that has several functions.

These seven constituents, also known as the cycle of nutrition, are:

1. Nutritional essence or *dang ma* (Tib. *dangs ma*) is connected to the process of mastication, digestion, and assimilation and formed by the nutrients we eat. Beginning in the mouth, we can chew food thanks to all-pervasive wind. We can taste through the tasting phlegm in the tongue, and produce saliva through the life-sustaining wind. The ascending wind allows swallowing and peristalsis of the esophagus. In the stomach, the mixing phlegm and the fire accompanying wind perform the work of breaking down food components, dividing them into more digestible constituents.

When the food reaches the small intestine, the digestive bile and fire accompanying wind separate out the pure part (nutritional essence or *dang ma*) that nourishes the body and is directed to the liver. The unclean part then continues toward the large intestine where, through the descending wind, it will be eliminated from the body.

2. Blood or *trag* (Tib. *khrag*) transports all substances extracted from the nutritional essence by the liver, which recovers nutrition and distributes it to the cells. All this is due to the all-pervasive wind, which gives movement. Due to heat generated within the liver, the pure part of the nutritional essence is transformed into blood, while the impure part will form the bile in the gall bladder. Bile aids the decomposition of food in the digestive process.

3. Muscle tissue or *sha* (Tib. *sha*): Different types of muscle tissue, smooth and striated, allow the operation of most of our organ systems and voluntary movement. All this is supported by the all-pervasive wind, as well as the other winds. The pure essence becomes adipose tissue and cartilage, while the impure part will be eliminated through the nine orifices.

4. Fat or *tsil* (Tib. *tshil*) serves to support and protect internal organs and helps to store water and nutrients. The pure portion is converted into bone tissue, while the impure portion forms sweat and sebaceous secretions.

5. The bones or *ru* (Tib. *rus*) form the skeletal system, the supporting structure of the body. The bones allow for the maintenance of positions and guide movements, and therefore are responsible for one's relationship with the surrounding world. The pure portion becomes core/marrow, while the impure portion forms the hair, teeth, and nails.

6. Bone marrow or *kang* (Tib. *rKang*) contributes to the development of a good constitution and to the replacement of blood cells. The pure portion gives rise to the reproductive fluids and cells (sperm and egg), while the impure part becomes skin, excrement, and oily elements used by our body.

7. Reproductive fluids or *kuwa* (Tib. *khu ba*) allow reproductive function. According to subtle anatomy, the *kuwa* is transformed and the essence goes to the heart and can be seen in the radiance of the complexion. At the gross level the *kuwa* becomes the sperm and the ovum. The impure portion becomes seminal fluid and menstrual blood.

The three leaves on the third branch of the tree of health/balance represent the three excretions. Due to these it is possible to detoxify the body by eliminating catabolic waste and the waste products of digestion.

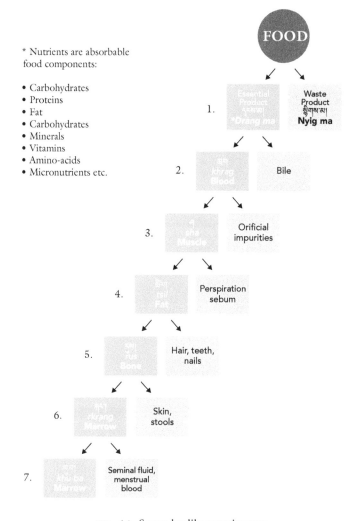

* Nutrients are absorbable
food components:

• Carbohydrates
• Proteins
• Fat
• Carbohydrates
• Minerals
• Vitamins
• Amino-acids
• Micronutrients etc.

FIG. 14. Seven bodily constituents

Feces are eliminated by the descending wind.

Urine is the product of elimination in the filtration process of the kidneys. If we ingest adequate amounts of fluids (water, teas, etc.) and the descending wind is in equilibrium, we eliminate urine, avoiding excess fluid and expelling the products that could cause imbalance.

Perspiration has to do with the all-pervasive wind that favors the expansion of the pores, together with the complexion-clearing bile allowing the formation and excretion of sweat. Perspiring is also a way to purify the skin, an important organ of the body, which must be clear and hydrated to stay healthy.

The three excretions represent the final part of the cycle of nutrition. Our health depends on how and what we eat. For this reason, nutrition comes first in the above list, and everything else derives from that. We should avoid ingesting the poison of excessive amounts of alcohol, sugar, and processed and refined foods. Furthermore, if we have a healthy body, physically and energetically, our children will also be healthy, because as with genetics in allopathic medicine, Sowa Rigpa considers that we inherit some of our tendencies from our parents.

Mental Balance

At the top of the trunk of health/balance are two flowers and three fruits. The two flowers are "long life," called *tse ring* (Tib. *tse ring; ring* means long and *tse* lifetime), and "good health," called *ne mey* (Tib. *nad med; med* means no and *nad* disease). These can flourish when the fifteen energies derived from the three humors are in balance, the seven constituents work well, the three excretions are disposed of without difficulty, and we are physically and mentally in good health. And as a result, we can achieve a long life.

The flowers are necessary in order for the fruits of mind to develop. In this context Sowa Rigpa philosophy resembles the Latin proverb "*mens sana in corpore sano*," which translates as "a healthy mind in a healthy body." The fruits are the three desirable mental states in Tibetan medicine: dharma, *chö* (Tib. *chos*); wealth, *nor* (Tib. *nor*); happiness, *de wa* (Tib. *de ba*).

Dharma (which translates as "law of all phenomena") or dharma mind means to be gifted with a pure mind, which arises with the proper attitude toward life and the ability to understand the true reality of things.

Dharma does not necessarily refer to those who practice the Buddhist philosophy. Anyone can have a mind that experiences the world in a "natural way," quietly and without opposing anything or creating conflicts. One deeply understands that events occur through causes and conditions that are present, not because life is revolting against one. If on a mental and emotional level we can accept what is happening, or at least experience it without too much tension, certainly we live better. This consciousness is needed to attain mental balance in life.

Wealth in this context does not simply mean money and possessions. Wealth is the result of a balanced mind. If the mind isn't balanced, we can possess anything and everything, but we will always crave more!

There is a story that expresses this concept very well. One day, a Tibetan lama visited the Chinese emperor, who claimed to be the richest man in China and listed proudly all his wealth. The emperor asked the lama who was the richest person in Tibet and what he possessed. The lama at first did not know what to say. After thinking for a while, he said that the richest man in the world possessed nothing, lived in a cave, and was named Milarepa, one of the foremost masters of Tibetan Buddhism.[1] The emperor did not understand why he had nothing, yet was considered the wealthiest person in Tibet. The lama replied that he was rich in the mind and therefore did not lack anything in life.

Happiness is what we all aspire to and the final goal in our life. We can experience happiness with material wealth and possessions, but it is brief and fleeting. True happiness comes from a dharma mind that understands the true nature of self and all phenomena and a pure mind that is contented and not craving more. Happiness can be achieved by both material and spiritual wealth, and the basis for this is good health.

The point of Tibetan medicine is to achieve and maintain balance in the three humors, seven constituents, and three excretions, so that the two flowers of long life and good health will grow and produce the fruits of dharma, wealth, and happiness. But when imbalances occur, these flowers will be stunted so that long life and good health are absent, and the fruits of dharma, wealth, and happiness cannot ripen. This balance should touch every level—energy, body, and mind. We will explore how imbalance occurs in the next chapter.

---

[1] Milarepa (*Rje-btsun Mi-la-ras-pa*) (1051–1135), one of the foremost masters of the Kagyu school of Tibetan Buddhism. Through extraordinary effort, he overcame his hardships from younger days and with the help of his master, Marpa Lotsawa, devoted his life to solitary meditation. Due to his practice of *gtum mo* or mystic fire, Milarepa was dressed in rags and thin white cotton cloth and meditated mostly in the freezing caves of the Himalayas. Milarepa engaged in meditation with zeal and devotion to achieve complete enlightenment. Soon his fame spread and many people wanted to hear the sublime songs through which he expressed his achievement. In one of his spiritual songs, he sang: "I have no desire for wealth or possessions, and so I have nothing. I do not experience the initial suffering of having to accumulate possessions, the intermediate suffering of having to guard and keep up possessions, or the final suffering of losing the possessions."

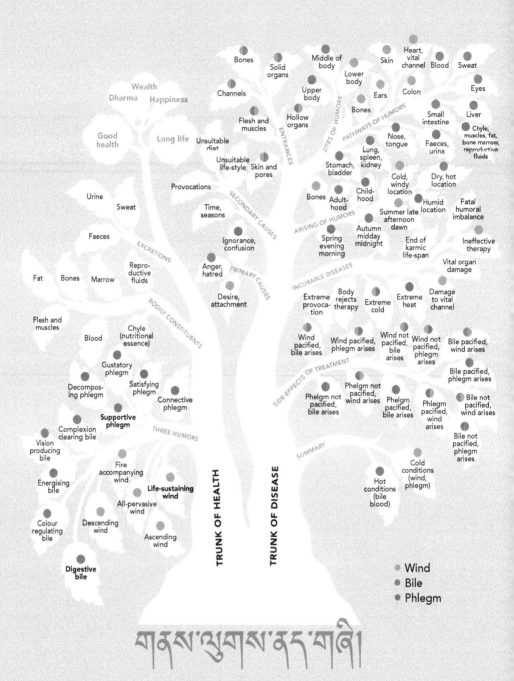

FIG. 15. The Tree of Health and Disease
Highlighting the Three Fruits and Two Flowers

5

The Origin of Imbalance

Chapter Outline

ROOTS OF DISEASE (2 TRUNKS)

I. Trunk of health (3 branches)
   A. Three humors (15 leaves)
      1. Wind/*loong*
      2. Bile/*tripa*
      3. Phlegm/*beken*
   B. Seven constituents (7 leaves)
   C. Three excretions (3 leaves)
   D. Two flowers and three fruits

II. Trunk of disease (9 branches)
   A. Primary causes (3 leaves)
   B. Secondary causes (4 leaves)
   C. Entrances (6 leaves)
   D. Sites of humors (3 leaves)
   E. Pathways of humors (15 leaves)
   F. Arising of humors (9 leaves)

G. Incurable diseases (9 leaves)
H. Side effects of treatment (12 leaves)
I. Summary (2 leaves)

Continuing on the tree of health and disease, the second trunk is the trunk of disease/imbalance. It has nine branches. The first branch represents the **primary causes** of imbalance. This branch has three leaves representing the three mental poisons (Tib. *dug sum*), desire, anger, and ignorance. At times, pride and envy are included, making five mental poisons.

The mental poisons/emotions do not directly cause disease, but they create the conditions for it. They are also called long-distance causes or indirect causes. For example, if someone likes to eat sweets, desire makes them eat more and can damage their health, causing overweight, diabetes, or metabolic problems. The same is true of drinking alcohol excessively, smoking, or any other habit that causes us to live a lifestyle in which attachment or other mental poisons/emotions prevail. If we nurture too much desire and attachment, we are led to do things excessively. We have so many ideas or

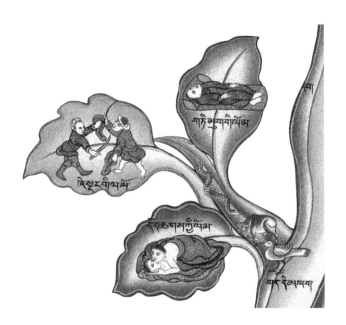

FIG. 16. The three poisons of mind:
desire, anger, and ignorance

thoughts that our mind is agitated and tired. This may cause a disorder of wind/*loong*. If aversion is excessive, if we develop a lot of anger, it can manifest a disorder of bile/*tripa*. Being lazy about mental and physical health can increase intellectual confusion and lead to a disorder of phlegm/*beken*.

In Tibetan, the term *dug sum* does not have an exclusively negative value. It indicates a hazardous substance that, if used in the correct way and in the correct amount, can be beneficial. Otherwise it may cause damage. Hazardous substances can be good medicine too. For example, aconite consumed without preparation and excessively can be poisonous and harmful. But taken in small doses after preparations like boiling and mixing with other substances, it is beneficial. Likewise for nutmeg, a very common spice that can be a dangerous poison if taken excessively but in the correct amount can be a good medicine. With mental poisons/emotions, we cannot say we are completely free. For example, having anger is normal and in the right amount can be a medicine too. The five poisons can be processed, or at least mitigated, by the five primordial wisdoms that express the pure and positive aspects of the mind. Poison and wisdom can be considered as two sides of a coin, or the latter as the antidote to the former. If we learn that some of these poisons predominate in us, we can meditate on the corresponding primordial wisdom and thus mitigate the negative effects.

The five wisdoms are five mental states attributed to the Dharmakaya, the realization of the subtle mind, and are represented by the five Dhyani buddhas. A Tibetan medicine practitioner can use this knowledge to give patients suggestions on how to work with their emotions, transforming mental poisons into wisdom mind.

The **secondary causes** (on the second branch) of disease are diet, the seasons, negative influences, and behavior.

TABLE 5.1

The five poisons and the five primordial wisdoms

POISON	PRIMORDIAL WISDOM
Pride	Wisdom of equanimity
Ignorance	Reality wisdom or state of phenomena wisdom
Attachment	Discriminating wisdom
Jealousy and envy	Wisdom that leads to achievement
Anger or disgust	Mirrorlike wisdom

Diet

There are two aspects to diet: quantity and quality. We tend to eat too much, largely due to the influence of the media. False advertising creates false desire, which leads to rampant consumption and unhealthy eating habits. In a day, with all the meals and snacks—breakfast, lunch, dinner, and several small meals in between—we may ingest enough food to nourish several people. More and more people are coming to this realization and are choosing to adopt a balanced approach to their consuming habits. Sowa Rigpa has proposed and promoted these principles for centuries. At the mercy of desires, due to emotional needs and stress, following fashion trends, and being influenced by subconscious advertising, we spend too much and consume more than necessary, with probable repercussions on health and wasting important resources.

The Seasons

Particular humors are associated with each season,[1] each time of day, each age range, and weather and climate patterns. For Sowa Rigpa, any period of time, any moment, assumes a precious significance because it is connected to a certain humor or energy.

TABLE 5.2
The humors and their connections with time, age, and seasons

PREVALENCE	LOONG	TRIPA	BEKEN
Hours	4–7 a.m. and 4–7 p.m.	midnight–3 a.m. and noon–3 p.m.	8–11 a.m. and 8–11 p.m.
Season	Summer	Autumn	Spring
Age	Over 70	Between 16 and 70	Under 16
Locality	Cold and windy	Hot and dry	Humid and cold

[1] Here it is done in reference also to the contents of the sixth branch, which indicates the times of growth of the three humors.

The pathologies caused by wind/*loong* are predominant during summer, in the afternoon and at dawn. The imbalances of bile/*tripa* increase in autumn, around noon, and at midnight. The diseases due to phlegm/*beken* are more frequent in the spring, early in the morning, and at the end of the day.

A cold and windy environment increases wind/*loong*, while places that are hot and closed in are unfavorable for bile/*tripa* and humid localities increase phlegm/*beken*.

Older people (over the age of 70) can develop pathologies connected to wind/*loong* changes, adults (16 to 70) are more prone to diseases caused by imbalances of bile/*tripa*, and children and teenagers (under 16) are prone to phlegm/*beken* imbalances.

Negative Influences

In Tibetan culture it is believed that by mistreating nature and polluting the environment, we disturb the spirits living there. These entities can revolt and cause illnesses, known as provocations. However, according to Sowa Rigpa, provocations include microorganisms, like bacteria and viruses, as well as mental beliefs in negative energies and harmful emotions. While Sowa Rigpa does not have the categories of viruses and bacteria, often illnesses caused by them are considered provocations from the spirits. There are different classifications of harmful spirits that can cause these problems, but in Tibetan medicine they are mainly classified according to elements and colors, with the disease having a connection with nature. These spirits dwell in lakes, rivers, oceans, and mountains. For example, *lu dud* (Tib. *klu bdud*, Skt. *naga*) are water spirits that can be found in springs, lakes, rivers, oceans, etc. They are tranquil beings, sending provocations like skin diseases, leprosy, and swelling in the limbs only if the water where they live is polluted or diverted. *Tsan* (Tib. *dtsan*) are very strong and quick-tempered spirits with aggressive and dangerous power that dwell in mountainous regions. These spirits provoke intense heart attacks and strokes with very acute and unexpected pain. Most of the elemental spirits are positive spirits who protect nature, sending provocations only when humans provoke or incite their wrathfulness with negative actions. In recent times, these provocations are more prominent due to air pollution, water pollution, excessive digging of the earth, and excessive use of chemicals. Therefore, in Sowa Rigpa, environmental and ecology issues are important for our balance and well-being. Through a deeper understanding of nature and elemental spirits, we can make more conscious choices and bring more peace and balance to our lives.

Lifestyle

Lifestyle in Sowa Rigpa has a huge and fundamental importance, and is very broad in scope. The proper amount and quality of sleep, physical exercise, work, rest, and even sex make a difference for your health. Keeping a healthy balance on the mental level is also important. One must avoid excesses not only of substances such as alcohol, food, and cigarettes, but also in the mind and in the contemplative process. If we spend too much time meditating but forget to move, our mind can become powerful but our physical body will suffer and manifest pathologies.

But it is not enough just to have the right diet. According to Sowa Rigpa, it is also necessary to behave responsibly by avoiding excesses and living with the interdependency principle in mind at all times. The interdependency principle calls upon each of us to reflect on the work done by all sentient beings (from the farmer to the seller) and to show gratitude for the ones that are sacrificed (animals, insects) for us to have food. By remembering that each part, each tissue, each cell of our body is dependent upon the external world, we give thanks for the well-being of everyone connected to us, whether they are close or distant. We are connected to our environment, and through mindfulness we can live with less stress and anger.

How Imbalances Enter the Body

In the part of the tree concerning the pathologies, the third branch (third from the left, counting from the bottom) shows the **entryway of imbalance**:

1. Propagation through skin
2. Diffusion into the muscular tissue
3. Circulation in the interior of the vessels and channels
4. Propagation through the bone tissue

5. Penetration into the solid organs
6. Penetration inside the hollow organs

Concentration of Humors in the Body

The next branch with three leaves indicates where the humors are concentrated in the body. The upper part of the body, the forehead and the shoulders, is the primary location of phlegm/*beken* energy; the central part, between the shoulders and the navel, is where bile/*tripa* prevails; the area from the navel down to the feet is the home of wind/*loong*. Knowing this distribution is useful when a practitioner gathers the medical history, observing the body and keeping in mind where the preponderance of signs and symptoms are located, to help formulate a diagnosis.

Circulatory Pathways of the Humors

The next branch of the tree represents the circulatory pathways of pathology according to the humors, located in the body constituents, sense organs, impurities of the body, solid organs, and hollow organs. In a wind/*loong* disease, the symptoms show in the bones, the ears, the skin and hair, the heart, and the large intestine. If the disease is bile/*tripa* in nature, traces in the blood are revealed in the eyes, the perspiration, the liver, the gall bladder, and the small intestine. Phlegm/*beken* diseases manifest in the chyle, muscles, fat, medulla, reproductive fluids, nose and tongue, feces and urine, lungs, spleen, kidneys, stomach, and urinary bladder.

Incurable Diseases

The branch of the **incurable or karmic diseases**[2] is on the right, the third from the bottom. These are due to:

---

[2] Some diseases cannot be cured completely, and there are nine incurable diseases in the Tibetan medicine text, as indicated. There are parallels in Western medicine, for example, injury to vital organs like the lungs, heart, or brain as well as extremely strong inflammation and infections.

1. Exhaustion of the three karmic factors of lifespan, merit, and past actions that sustain life

2. Fatal combinations of hot and cold pathologies

3. Treatment of disease with the wrong medicine, i.e., using medicine of an identical nature to the disease

4. Injury to the vulnerable points or vital organs of the body

5. Delay in treating a pathology of the ascending wind, which involves the three main factors: breathing, heartbeat, and brain activity

6. Delay in treating feverish conditions

7. Delay in curing a pathology of cold nature that allows the cold to penetrate the body and become profoundly ingrained

8. Exhaustion of the body constituents that does not respond to treatments

9. Extreme injury resulting in the loss of the *la*,[3] due to a provocation from the elemental spirits, *lu dud,* or others.

In these cases, the practitioner mainly provides support, helping the person to accept the disease and prepare for their subsequent death. The doctor stays next to the person, preparing them progressively for this unavoidable event, working toward acceptance of the situation and helping them face the fear that may accompany it.

Tibetan doctors do not refuse to care for a patient with an incurable disease just because there are no treatments capable of curing them, but support them, helping them keep a positive mind. This attitude is very useful also to the therapist, increasing his professional and spiritual growth.

---

[3] *La* (Tib. *bLa*) in Tibetan means superior body or energy body. Between the physical body and the mind, the *la* is an energetic copy of the physical body. It is fundamental to connection of the body and the mind and is one aspect of harmony and well-being between them. Therefore *la* imbalances can cause a profound imbalance of the physical constituents and the mind. The *la* channel flows from the heart through the ulnar artery to the attachment of the annular ligaments of the fingers. For this reason, in the external therapy of *Kunye*, Tibetan massage, a red thread is placed on the base of the fourth fingers and toes to protect the *la*. Some spirits, when they cannot attack the physical body, take hold of the *la*. A body deprived of this energy is likely to be stripped of its vital essence and therefore is in a very dangerous situation. (*La* will be explained more extensively in chapter 8 under external therapies.)

The next branch (on the bottom, the second from the right) represents disease produced as a side effect of or reaction to the therapy itself. These byproducts of the therapy manifest when:

1. Wind/*loong* is brought into balance, but a bile/*tripa* imbalance arises
2. Wind/*loong* is stabilized, but a phlegm/*beken* instability arises
3. Bile/*tripa* is put into balance, but wind/*loong* energy is changed
4. Bile/*tripa* is stabilized, but phlegm/*beken* is imbalanced
5. Phlegm/*beken* is rebalanced, but a bile/*tripa* alteration occurs
6. The treatment of wind/*loong* excess is not effective and a bile/*tripa* change manifests
7. The treatment of wind/*loong* disorder is not effective and a phlegm/*beken* imbalance is created
8. The treatment of bile/*tripa* disorder is not effective and a wind/*loong* imbalance is created
9. The treatment of bile/*tripa* imbalance is not effective and a phlegm/*beken* imbalance is created
10. The treatment of phlegm/*beken* disorder is not effective and a wind/*loong* imbalance is created
11. The treatment of phlegm/*beken* imbalance is not effective and a bile/*tripa* imbalance is created.

The last branch on the bottom summarizes by categorizing diseases into two classes: those that are hot conditions or *tsawa*, which is related to blood and bile/*tripa*, and those that are cold conditions or *drangwa*, which is related to wind/*loong* and phlegm/*beken*.

With this knowledge of the tree of health and disease, i.e., what is balance, what is imbalance and how, when, and where disease arises, in the next chapter, we will look at the next root: the tree of diagnosis.

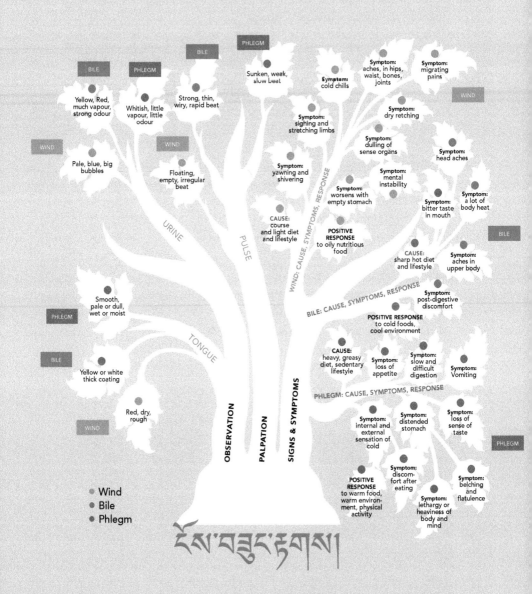

FIG. 17. The Tree of Diagnosis

6

The Art of Diagnosis

Chapter Outline

III. Trunk of medical history (3 branches)
 A. Wind/*loong* medical history (1 leaf)
 B. Bile/*tripa* medical history (1 leaf)
 C. Phlegm/*beken* medical history (1 leaf)

Diagnosis is of major importance in Sowa Rigpa, as in any other medical discipline. All treatment starts with diagnosis—though traditional Tibetan medicine (TTM) diagnoses must not be confused with those of any other medical system, as there is no one-to-one correspondence between the diagnostic systems. For example, a patient with an allopathic diagnosis of migraine headaches may have any one of several TTM diagnoses. And the reverse is also true: a patient with the TTM diagnosis of phlegm/*beken* imbalance may have the allopathic diagnoses of indigestion, sinusitis, or depression.

It is indispensable to know the patient's typology, that is, the normal physiological composition of humors/energetic principles in their body, as well as their pathology, that is, the disease they are suffering from. Only with correct diagnosis can one apply the correct remedy. The physician must understand the patient's symptoms and the underlying functions of the body systems and use this information to develop a treatment plan.

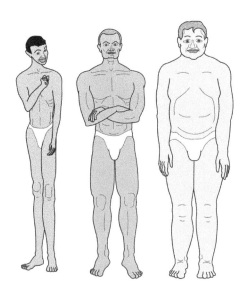

FIG. 18. Humoral Typology

Humoral Typology Test

To understand the humoral typology of an individual, it is necessary to determine which energy is predominant in them.

While this is in no way a substitution for thorough evaluation by a well-trained Tibetan doctor, the following test can help one organize the signs and symptoms of the three humors and determine which is most prevalent. It is possible that two or three humors may all be prevalent depending on the balance of signs and symptoms.

The three main tools a Sowa Rigpa practitioner uses to determine the diagnosis are observation, palpation, and diagnostic questioning.

TABLE 6.1
Humoral typology test

CHARACTERISTICS	WIND/LOONG	BILE/TRIPA	PHLEGM/BEKEN
Structure	Little; thin; tendency to kyphosis	Medium; erect posture, open chest; athletic, physical	Voluminous; strong muscles; erect posture
Complexion	Olive color; dry and rough	Yellowish; oily	Light; soft and hydrated
Hair	Dry	Greasy	Heavy and hydrated
Body temperature	Sensitive to cold	Hot	Cold
Articulations	Salient and cracking	Normal	Hidden
Mind aspects	Agile mind, in constant movement; ment; concentration difficulty; short-term memory; openness to the new	Sharp and fast mind; strong intuition; analytic intelligence; strong self-esteem	Calm mind; mental stability; slow thinking; mental laziness; slow acceptance of the new; long-term memory
Emotions	Emotionality; extroversion; emotional instability; impatience	Combativeness; pride; jealousy; competitiveness; egocentrism	Gentleness; patience; tolerance; passivity; humility; emotional balance
Temperament	Nervous, active, and combative; great imagination; sensitive; anticonformist	Easily irritable; communicative; assertive; motivated and sure about goals; tendency to obsessiveness	Tranquil, quiet; reliable and understandable; persevering; slow and monotonous; tendency to conformism

The Art of Diagnosis

CHARACTERISTICS	WIND/LOONG	BILE/TRIPA	PHLEGM/BEKEN
Common problems	Lower part of the body; tensions and muscular spasms; constipation; rapid skin aging; premature aging	Upper part of the body; eye problems; tendency to baldness; headache; nausea	Difficult and slow digestion; stomach pains after meals; feeling of internal cold; slow blood circulation
Sleep	Light and insufficient; fragmented dreams; tendency to awake in the middle of the night; tendency to insomnia	Normal; vivid dreams; tendency to awake in the middle of the night; easily awakened in the morning	Profound; heavy; abundant; difficulty awakening in the morning
Digestion	Variable metabolism; tendency to eat irregularly; loses weight easily, gains with difficulty	Intense metabolism; constant weight; no digestive problems	Slow metabolism; regular appetite; gains weight easily, loses with difficulty
Favorite taste	Salty, sweet, sour, bitter	Sweet, bitter, blunt, astringent	Spicy, sour, astringent, salty
Metaphor	Vulture, crow, fox	Tiger, monkey[1]	Elephant[2]
Tongue	Dry; red; reddish tip; rough	Thick yellow-and-white coating; red edges; bitter taste in mouth	Pallid; whitish; soft; moist
Pulse	Fluctuates[3];empty[4]; irregular beat	Full[5]; tense[6]; rapid beat	Profound[7]; slow beat
Urine	Clear like water or bluish; irregular stream; weak odor; large bubbles	Yellow or red; a lot of steam; intense odor; medium bubbles that disappear rapidly; lots of sediment	Clear, whitish, grayish; no steam; no odor; small bubbles, similar to foam, that remain for a long time

---

[1] An animal with large energetic capacity and a lot of initiative.

[2] A calm animal, stable and with good memory.

[3] Like an air bubble in a tube.

[4] Superficially palpable, vanishes with increased pressure.

[5] Like a tube full of water, easy to touch, difficult to compress.

[6] Like a rope under tension.

[7] It has to be pressed to be detected.

Observation

The practitioner looks to collect as much information as possible to make a precise diagnosis. He or she observes the general aspect of the patient like how they move, talk, take care of themselves, etc.; observes the color and the skin condition, the nose, and the tongue; evaluates the urine; examine the eyes and ears; feels the pulse; moves joints to confirm functional limitations and observe the pain due to movement. Through palpation the practitioner observes the extent of the edema, swelling, clicking, and deformation of the articulation. One has to listen to the patient very carefully, cultivating an attitude of deep respect, seeking to understand the most profound substance of what is being communicated without conceit and any preconceived notions of what may be wrong with the patient's health.

More specifically, observation is done in a focused way concerning the tongue, eyes, aspect and exterior characteristics of the body, nose, and ears.

Tongue Diagnosis

As mentioned in chapter 3, there is a direct relationship between organs and body parts, and they can be represented as parts of a flower; the solid organ is the root or seed, the hollow organ is the stem, and the sense organs are the flower, the part that is manifested. When evaluating a patient, using the schematic representation of the flower, we can infer the conditions of internal organs.

As a flower organ, the tongue can give conclusive information about the small intestines (stem) and heart (root organ) in general. For example, the tip of the tongue will appear red when there is an excess of heat in the heart. And the color, aspect, and surface of the tongue can indicate a humoral imbalance.

For a person in good health, the tongue is red in color and soft, moist, and mobile.

The tongue in a person with wind/*loong* imbalance is reddish, dry, and rough, with a thick blue vein underneath.

The tongue in a person with bile/*tripa* imbalance has a thick yellowish or whitish coating with a dirty aspect to it. The patient often says that they have a bitter taste in their mouth.

The tongue in a person with phlegm/*beken* imbalance has a grayish coating with mucus and is sticky, with a soft surface. Sometimes it can be swollen, as evidenced by teeth marks on the sides.

Eye Diagnosis

Although examination of the eyes is not considered a primary method of diagnosis, such observation helps to confirm the diagnosis. As a flower organ, the eyes can give distinctive information on the gall bladder (stem) and liver (root organ). For example, if the eyes are dry and the veins are full of blood, this indicates an excess of heat in the bile or blood. And black dots at the end of a vein in the eye denote the presence of chronic bile disease in the liver or gall bladder. The eyes can also give information on humoral nature or imbalance.

Eyes that show wind/*loong* nature are small, with a direct look, and nervous; there are few eyelashes, the eyelids are a little flaccid, and the sclera a little opaque. The gaze is fixed; the iris can be dark with a gradient between gray and brown, or dark, and the eyes blink often. If there is a *loong* disorder the sclera can be red.

Eyes that show bile/*tripa* nature are of medium size, penetrating, and bright. They are sensitive to light. The iris can be permeated with yellow or red, as can the sclera. In cases of *tripa* disorders the ocular surface can be yellow and blood vessels can be seen.

Eyes that show phlegm/*beken* nature are big and beautiful, moist, with long eyelashes, thick and oily. The iris has very bright colors and can be a little swollen. In case of a *beken* disorder the sclera can be pale and the patient may complain of reduced vision.

Nose Diagnosis

The nose is the flower organ of the colon (stem organ) and lungs (root organ). Knowing how to read the signs and symptoms detectable through the nose helps to circumscribe the diagnosis more precisely.

The nose that is sniffing indicates little energy in the lungs, or excess phlegm/*beken* in the head.

If the nose is irritated or has purulent inflammation, this can be a sign of a cold, influenza, or an allergic reaction.

A patient reporting obstructed or dry nose may have a pulmonary disorder.

The presence of a dark pimple on the nose tip is a sign of pathology at the digestive system level.

The presence of pus and frequent sneezing indicates a chronic disease in the interior of the body.

Excessive facial oil around the nostrils shows excess heat at the spleen and liver level.

Ear Diagnosis

The ears are the flower of the urinary bladder and kidneys. By analyzing the ears, we can assess the physical and energetic conditions of the organs as well the mental condition of the individual. Ear diagnosis is useful especially with infants and children, because it is often very difficult to diagnose the conditions of their organs through pulse reading;[8] a child's pulse is fainter than an adult's and can be very fast. Therefore, it is better to observe the paths of the veins in the ears, as they are very similar to the paths of the arteries in the circulatory system. Using natural light or a small flashlight, placed in the anterior part of the ear, three blood vessels are visible; each corresponds to an internal organ. In the presence of an excess wind/*loong* disorder, such veins become clearer.

---

[8] Pulse reading can be found in all traditions of oriental medicine like Chinese medicine, Indian Ayurvedic medicine, and of course, Tibetan medicine. They are all ancient systems, each with its own specific characteristics and historical background. Tibetan pulse checking is a very old science, mentioned in several ancient medical texts along with several spiritual practices. Pulse reading is another unique diagnostic method, next to urine analysis. The extent of its variety, sensibility, and quality cannot be found in other traditional medical systems.

TABLE 6.2
Scheme of the ear blood vessels

BLOOD VESSEL	RIGHT EAR MEN	LEFT EAR MEN	RIGHT EAR WOMEN	LEFT EAR WOMEN
Superior	Lungs	Heart	Heart	Lungs
Medium	Liver	Spleen	Liver	Spleen
Inferior	Right kidney	Left kidney	Right kidney	Left kidney

Diagnosis of the Physical Constitution

Analyzing the height, complexion, and body structure of the patient provides useful information for establishing the kind of treatment to prescribe.

Physical aspects of a wind/*loong* person: dark complexion, skinny, fragile, short, dry and cold skin.

Physical aspects of a bile/*tripa* person: yellowish complexion, blond/light-colored hair, medium height, sweats a lot, oily and hot skin.

Physical aspects of a phlegm/*beken* person: erect posture, tendency to excess weight, slow movement, round face, oily skin, soft and cold.

Urine Diagnosis

Urine analysis probably has its roots in the shamanic practice of the pre-Buddhist Bon culture. At that time, it was considered an art or divinatory type of practice, used to identify provocations. This ancient art continues today in its entirety, making Tibetan medicine unique among the healing traditions. Examining the urine is very important, as it gives information directly from the body. Therefore, it is said that the urine is the mirror of the internal body.

There are three points of time and ten characteristics of the urine that should be examined. The three time points are when the urine is warm, tepid, and cold. While the urine is warm, the practitioner should observe the color, steam, odor, and bubbles. When the urine is tepid, one should observe the sediment and the coating. Finally, when the urine is cold, one should note the time of transformation, the way that it is transformed, color, and viscosity. Ideally, the practitioner should observe the urine at all three time points.

To allow for a precise observation, the patient must follow some guidelines concerning food and behavior prior to the collection of the liquid. The patient must avoid drugs or drinks that can change the color; alcohol, which increases bile properties; spicy, salty, and fatty foods; large amounts of raw food; and fizzy drinks. Furthermore, the person must have a regular night of sleep, have a calm mind, avoid sexual intercourse, avoid drinking anything after midnight, and urinate before going to sleep.

The urine for analysis is the first of the morning, which should be placed in a clean container made of glass, white porcelain, enameled steel, or adequate metal. Materials like clay, copper, and brass should be avoided.

The urine of a person in good health has a yellow color like straw, tending toward amber; a light odor; steam (usually found on the walls of the closed container) of moderate intensity, uniform and tending to disappear slowly. The bubbles or the foam that forms after agitating vigorously are of a medium size and quantity and do not disappear rapidly. When the container is left closed, uniform sediment forms that is not consistent. The revetment or oily coating found on the surface when the urine cools off is difficult to detect. Finally, the urine changes color, becoming clear and clean as it cools.

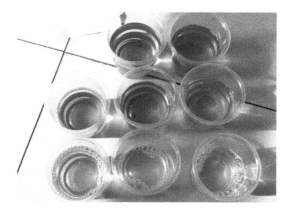

FIG. 19. Urine analysis in a Tibetan hospital in Xining, Amdo

The urine of a person with an imbalance of one or more humors can present the following characteristics:

Wind/*loong* disorders: as with all things influenced by wind, the characteristics change rapidly and are irregular. While the urine is hot, the coloration is bluish and transparent, similar to fountain water; the steam is distributed in a random manner and the odor intensity changes easily. When agitated, light bubbles form with a bluish tint and disappear rapidly one after another. When the urine is tepid and left to settle, the sediment is not abundant and forms hairlike filaments. The revetment is irregular. The time that the urine of a person with *loong* imbalance takes to cool off and change color is not always the same. The urine cools and changes color from the center to the periphery or the other way around, depending on the case. The final color is clear in some parts and turbid in others, with a bluish cast.

Bile/*tripa* disorders: while warm, the coloration is an intense yellow that can even be orange or red; the steam is abundant. The internal surface of the receptacle is cloudy, with condensation. The odor is fetid and pungent. If agitated, the liquid forms medium-sized bubbles that are yellowish and disappear rapidly, sometimes make a cracking noise. While the urine is still tepid, the sediment is copious, all diffuse in the form of snowflakes or clouds. The revetment that is formed is thick and oily. This liquid tends to cool off and to change color rapidly (around five minutes), clearing from the center to the periphery. When it is cold, this kind of urine becomes turbid and yellow.

Phlegm/*beken* disorders: while warm, the coloration is light yellow, with a tendency toward white, and the liquid can be turbid. The steam is not visible. There is no particular odor. Bubbles can be present. When agitated, small bubbles form that are stable, white, and sticky, similar to mucus, and disappear very slowly. When the liquid is tepid, the sediment is scarce, punctiform; the revetment is thin or absent. The cooling is very slow (more than five minutes) and the color change is verified at the end. As the urine cools, the color changes from the periphery to the center. When cold, the urine is clear, whitish, and transparent, with a small amount of sediment at the bottom.

Generally, if the urine has an odor of food substances, that means that the patient is having digestive difficulties or issues of absorption. The presence of abundant sediment, whatever the aspect, indicates excess bile. If the urine is cloudy, it indicates that the patient overeats. The absence of sediment generally indicates excess cold.

Palpation

Ancient Western physicians could give a precise diagnosis from examining the pulse. But this subtle art has been replaced by purely quantitative measurements, which are the emphasis of modern science. Modern Western doctors examine only the frequency and rhythm of the pulse, mainly to determine the condition of the heart. Similarly, in modern Western medicine the term "palpation" is reserved for touching the exterior of the body to feel the texture, size, and form of inner organs or tumors.

In Tibetan medicine, diseases of the inner organs are mainly diagnosed by indirect observation such as examination of the sense organs, urine analysis, and pulse reading. So, in Tibetan medicine, the term "palpation" is mainly used for pulse diagnosis. This technique is believed to have come from the pre-Buddhist Bon tradition, part of a very ancient cultural system that may date back to the ancient kingdom of Shang Shung, known as the cradle of Bon. In the *Bum Shi* (the first ancient text on Tibetan medicine), there is an entire chapter dedicated to pulse reading. This text, which dates back 3,900 years, also contains explanations on divination that were typical of the ancient Bon culture.

Palpation consists of checking the pulse on three levels: physical, energetic, and spiritual. In Sowa Rigpa, it primarily refers to feeling the multiple pulses at the radial pulse, that is, the pulse in the artery at the wrist. According to Sowa Rigpa, we can detect several kinds of pulses, which correspond to physiological, seasonal, and pathological aspects of health. The physiological or healthy constitutional pulses can vary according to the type of prevailing energy of wind, bile, and phlegm. The pulse is also affected by the seasons. And an unhealthy (pathological) pulse is distinguished through the frequency of the pulsation, which denotes a hot or cold condition.

Learning the physical aspects of taking pulse is very easy. Learning the energetic level takes more training, and the spiritual level takes much more training and a specific meditative retreat. More than just developing sensitivity of the fingers, the training also concerns developing spiritual qualities. Traditional Tibetan medicine texts recommend that practitioners go on a retreat[9] especially for the purpose of perfecting the art of taking pulses, to gain a deeper understanding of and ability to know the bioenergetics of the patient.

Theoretically, it is possible to detect the pulses of the twelve major organs of the body and so receive information about them. This is possible because wind together with blood circulate in the whole body, where they combine with the essential nutritive constituents. The pulsing movement that goes through the arteries, arrives at the organs, and from there makes a return beat is a movement, like a message, that can be deciphered by the practitioner's fingers. For example, if the heart-space-fire component is in excess, this is shown in a pulsation that is faster and more tense than normal. According to Sowa Rigpa, the diagnosis will be an excess of bile/*tripa* energy in the heart, energy that is associated with the space and fire elements.

The reading is done by using three fingers, index, middle, and ring finger, with attention given to either the right side or the left side of each fingertip. The pulses on the left and right radial arteries are taken at exact locations, each corresponding to a particular solid or hollow organ. This evaluation can be done on any artery of the body, but by convention and ease of access, the radial artery is the most commonly used.

For the most precise reading, the pulse should be taken two days in a row, just like the urine examination.

The patient's arm should be placed in a comfortable position. With men, the practitioner initiates the palpation in the left arm and takes the pulse with the right hand. With women, it is the other way around.

When reading a man's pulse, from the left:

Index finger: the left side of the fingertip detects the heart energy, the right side the small intestine energy

Middle finger: the left side detects the spleen energy, the right side the stomach energy

---

[9] The *Yuthok Nyingthig*, the text for the spiritual practice of Tibetan medicine, gives special instructions for pulse reading, addressed to physicians of traditional Tibetan medicine in particular. This technique is linked to both ordinary medical practice and spiritual practice. In this text, there is an entire practice of pulse checking through meditation. In a spiritual retreat practitioners can enhance their pulse diagnosis abilities through the blessings of medicine goddesses and rishis.

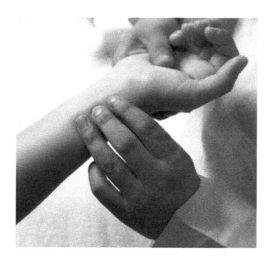

FIG. 20. Pulse reading

Ring finger: the left side detects the energetic condition of the left
    kidney, the right the condition of the genital organs.

When reading a man's pulse, on the right:

Index finger: the right side of the fingertip detects the lung energy,
    the left side the colon energy
Middle finger: the right side detects the liver energy, the left side the
    gall bladder energy
Ring finger: the right side detects the energy of the right kidney, the
    left side that of the urinary bladder.

When reading a woman's pulse, on the right:

Index finger: the right side of the fingertip detects the heart energy,
    the left side the small intestine energy
Middle finger: same as in men
Ring finger: same as in men.

When reading a woman's pulse, on the left:

The Art of Diagnosis

Index finger: the left side of the fingertip detects the lungs' energy;
    the one on the right, the colon energy
Middle finger: same as in men
Ring finger: same as in men.

The reason for this inversion between the pulses of men and women is explained in the tantric texts and subtle anatomy. Although many traditions believe that men have mainly solar energy, in the studies of Tibetan subtle anatomy, the opposite is stated. In men, lunar energy dominates; it is connected with the left energy channel, *kyangma,* so the heart pulse is palpable on the left side. In women, the predominant energy is of solar nature, connected with the right energy channel, *roma,* and the heart pulse is therefore read on the right side.

The other organs, whether they are solid or hollow, are in the same position in both sexes.

The three physiological pulses are named for their characteristics. ("Masculine" and "feminine" here refer just to the character of the pulse, and aren't related to the patient's gender.)

TABLE 6.3

Relationships between the palpation zones of the pulse
and the organs of the body

	MEN			
	Left hand	*Right hand*		
	Left side of the finger	Right side of the finger	Left side of the finger	Right side of the finger
Index finger	Heart	Small intestine	Colon	Lung
Middle	Spleen	Stomach	Gall bladder	Liver
Ring	Left kidney	Genital organs	Bladder	Right kidney
	WOMEN			
	Left hand	*Right hand*		
	Left side of the finger	Right side of the finger	Left side of the finger	Right side of the finger
Index finger	Lung	Colon	Small intestine	Heart
Middle	Spleen	Stomach	Gall bladder	Liver
Ring	Left kidney	Genital organs	Bladder	Right kidney

Masculine pulse (*loong* pulse): the beat is large, rough, thick, and
   floating.
Feminine pulse (*tripa* pulse): the beat is thin, tense, and rapid.
Bodhisattva pulse or neutral (*beken* pulse): the pulsations are profound, long, light, and calm.

At birth, according to Sowa Rigpa, each person has one of the three
physiological pulses. (Over time, a person's pulse can change according
to changes in their constitution caused by diet and lifestyle.) Identifying
the type is the first stage of determining the diagnosis and subsequent
treatment. However, during the disease phase, it is often difficult to detect
the physiological pulse, as it can be confused with one of the three humor
pulses in a disorder or pathological pulse.

For pulse detection, it is important to keep in mind the astrological
elements of the year, month, and hour in which the examination is done,
as each part of the day is affected by a humor. (See the table on page XX in
chapter 5.) More important, however, is the seasonal influence. This is due
to the influences of the five external elements on the pulse; these change
according to the season of the year, as described above.

In virtue of the several characteristics of the seasons, days, and hours,
the external energies (see chapter 3) affect the internal ones. These influences are traditionally called "friends," "enemies," and "mother" or "son"
relationships. When the energies are the same they are called friends; when
opposed, they are enemies. When the energies nurture each other they are
called mother relationships, and when one energy is supporting another
it is called a son pulse.

The emotions of the patient also influence the pulse reading. If the
patient is agitated or preoccupied, a superficial reading of the pulses could
give wrong indications.

Medical History

The medical history is obtained by collecting information about the probable causes of the illness, symptoms, and reactions to diet and lifestyle. A
qualified doctor should be able to conclude a diagnosis with the information drawn through observation and palpation. Medical history can be
used to clarify or to confirm a diagnosis that has already been made. In

some cases it is necessary to get otherwise difficult-to-access information like the patient's condition before manifestation of an illness. The patient's answers about habits and circumstances help to distinguish between physiology and pathology. As mentioned earlier, disorders happen due to diet and behavior that is not appropriate for the person's underlying typology/constitution. Therefore, there are two major focuses of the history: determining the underlying constitution of the patient and understanding the causes of the imbalance, whether it be the patient's diet, behavior, or external conditions.

Wind/*loong* disorders are characterized by excessive yawning, chills, tremors, the need to stretch, pain that moves from site to site in the lower part of the body, vomiting on an empty stomach, dullness of the sense organs, mental instability, and stomach cramps. Patients will report that their symptoms worsen with an empty stomach. Due to the nature of wind, the symptoms improve after they eat oily and nutritious foods.

Patients report hot symptoms if they have a bile/*tripa* disorder. For example, they often report a bitter taste in the mouth, headache, a feeling of high body heat, and pain in the upper part of the body and abdominal postdigestive pains. These symptoms are aggravated during digestion while the food is in the small intestine. Bile imbalance can be caused by overconsumption of hot and spicy food and an incorrect lifestyle, like drinking alcohol; ingesting excessive amounts of vinegar, lamb, or mutton; sitting in the sun or in hot places for long periods of time; sudden movements or strenuous physical activities. These symptoms improve with a diet rich in fresh food and regular rest.

Patients with phlegm/*beken* disorders tend to have symptoms that are cool and damp. They report having little appetite; digestion difficulties; vomiting; loss of the sense of taste; feeling of heaviness in the stomach; belching; heavy, slow, and dull perceptions of the body and mind; feeling cold either internally or externally; and discomfort after eating. The symptoms get worse after eating. They improve with the ingestion of warm foods, being in warm places, and increased physical activity. Phlegm imbalance is due to overconsumption of heavy, greasy, and oily foods; a sedentary lifestyle; and remaining in cold and humid places for long periods of time.

The advantage of the medical history is the distinct verbal communication between physician and patient. This can help create trust. For beginning practitioners, it can be a useful tool to extract necessary information from the patient. The disadvantage is that not all patients can or want to describe their problems in the correct way and therefore may mislead the doctor. Therefore, a physician should build a professional level of verbal communication and mutual trust with patients in order to make a good diagnosis.

In summary, to make a diagnosis, the doctor observes the tongue, the urine, and the sense organs and checks the pain points. Then they check the pulse and ask questions about causes of problems, symptoms, and reactions to diet and lifestyle. A qualified Tibetan medicine doctor must be able to make a correct diagnosis independent of the patient's compliance. Traditionally it took many years, even longer than our standard modern medical course of study, to reach that level of skill.

Having learned about balance, imbalance, and diagnosis, in the next chapter we look at the third root: the tree of therapy, the methods of healing.

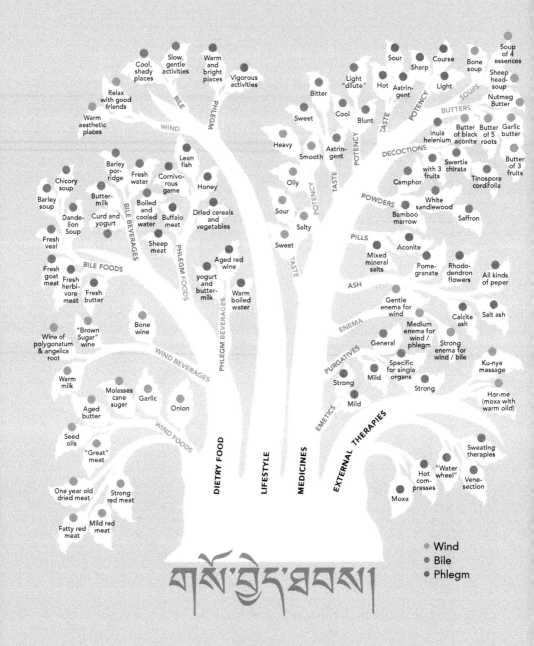

FIG. 20. The Tree of Therapies

7

A Natural Cure

Chapter Outline

ROOT OF TREATMENT METHOD (4 TRUNKS)

> A. Wind/*loong* food (10 leaves)
> B. Wind/*loong* drinks (4 leaves)
> C. Bile/*tripa* food (7 leaves)
> D. Bile/*tripa* drinks (5 leaves)
> E. Phlegm/*beken* food (6 leaves)
> F. Phlegm/*beken* drinks (3 leaves)
> II. Trunk of lifestyle (3 branches)
> > A. Wind/*loong* behavior (2 leaves)
> > B. Bile/*tripa* behavior (2 leaves)
> > C. Phlegm/*beken* behavior (2 leaves)
> III. Trunk of medicine (15 branches)
> > A. Wind/*loong* taste (3 leaves)
> > B. Wind/*loong* potency (3 leaves)

C. Bile/*tripa* taste (3 leaves)
D. Bile/*tripa* potency (3 leaves)
E. Phlegm/*beken* taste (3 leaves)
F. Phlegm/*beken* potency (3 leaves)
G. Soup (3 leaves)
H. Butter (5 leaves)
I. Decoction (4 leaves)
J. Powder (4 leaves)
K. Pill (2 leaves)
L. Ash (5 leaves)
M. Enema (3 leaves)
N. Laxative (4 leaves)
O. Emetic (2 leaves)

The *Four Tantras* describe the four basic methods of healing in Tibetan medicine: diet, lifestyle, herbal medicines, and external therapies. Healthy food and lifestyle are two of the most important factors in a healthy and long life and in the treatment of disorders. Once the disease has progressed to chronic stages, the practitioner needs to augment food and lifestyle recommendations with external therapies and herbal medicines. External therapies like massage, sweating treatment, moxa, and heat application will be described in subsequent chapters. In general, the practitioner should recommend dietary and lifestyle changes to increase the humors that are deficient and rebalance those that are in excess.

Diet and Lifestyle

Our health depends on how and what we eat and what we do. Since diet and behavior are two of the secondary causes of disease, changes of diet and behavior can help to cure the disease.

Reinforcing the concept of interdependence and interconnection, an ancient Tibetan proverb quoted in the *Four Tantras* says: "With the function of the five elements of food, the five element of the body will develop in balance." This means that keeping a good balance of internal elements depends on the intake of external elements. We are what we eat! Indeed, everything is derived from the five elements. Eating is the main way through which we incorporate them into our body. If we eat in a

CASE STUDY I

A patient, a French man who suffered from multiple sclerosis, had various symptoms including loss of clarity in vision due to an inflammation of the optic nerve. The disease was progressing and his symptoms were worsening. I recommended the Tibetan formula Gabur 25 (Camphor 25[1]) and some *nejang* yogic exercises for the eyes. After he followed the treatment for a few weeks, his symptoms began to stabilize and improve greatly. He continued with the herbal formula long term, and has been able to offset the progression of the disease.

healthy, balanced, and organic way, our five internal elements are balanced; if we eat food that is somehow unbalanced, this will lead to disorders in the internal elements. Health, disease, and treatment are of the same nature. The body is composed of five elements, the diseases are developed through the five elements, and treatment is based on the five elements.

CASE STUDY 2

Another patient, a French woman, had chronic eczema for ten years. She tried various types of creams, diet modifications, and other therapies, but nothing worked for long. I recommended that she do the ninefold purification breathing (Tib. *rlung ro bsal ba,* meaning expelling the dead wind), a meditative breathing exercise mentioned in chapter 3, for ten to fifteen minutes each day. Remarkably, her skin cleared up shortly after commencing the practice. The condition has not returned, and she maintains this as part of her daily meditation.

Simple breathing exercises incorporated into our daily lifestyle can have tremendous benefits for maintaining the balance and health of the body, energy, and mind.

---

[1] Traditional Tibetan medicine formulas are typically made from a variety of different natural substances. "Gabur 25" means a formula compounded from twenty-five substances with *gabur* or camphor as the main ingredient.

Tibetan medicine advises specific food and behavior according to the patient's typology or pathology. However, there are some rules that apply to all in order to maintain metabolic heat[2] and thus prevent complications connected with indigestion. For example, it is beneficial to start the day with a cup of hot water and to avoid overeating, especially in the evening when the metabolic heat is weak. Also avoid eating refined, processed foods and sugar, and drinking carbonated beverages.

Concerning behavior, more vigorous activities are suggested for phlegm/*beken* and gentle activities for wind/*loong* and bile/*tripa*. However, in the Tibetan medical tradition there is a special type of exercise that brings about perfect balance for everybody, regardless of their typology. It is called *nejang* (Tib. *gnas sbyangs*) and means cleansing the energy sites in the body. This healing method comes from the Kalachakra tradition and is a medical part of the Tibetan yoga, *tsaloong trulkor*, which is accessible also for untrained people. These special exercises use the power of breathing to unblock the energy flow in the body and thus remove the causes of problems. More description and instructions on the practice will be given below.

DIET AND LIFESTYLE RECOMMENDATIONS FOR
WIND/*LOONG* IMBALANCES

One should increase consumption of oily food (healthy fats) and nutrients like nuts and seeds, oils (especially sesame oil and old butter), grains, chicken, mutton, horse meat, salmon, sugarcane, molasses, garlic, and onion.

Drink hot milk, red sweet wine with sugarcane, barley beer, wheat beer with angelica root and tendril-leaf Solomon's seal, meat and bone broth, and hot drinks before and after meals.

---

[2] Metabolic heat or *medrod* is the basis of all digestive processes, the digestive bile in particular. It supplies heat to the humors, bodily constituents, and excretions. Metabolic heat ensures good health, energy, radiance of complexion, and long life. Strong digestive heat will ensure proper digestion and allow waste products to move downward for excretion. With weak digestive heat, food will not be digested properly and will pass undigested. Metabolic heat is the main factor responsible in the cycle of nutrition: synthesizing food into bodily constituents, ensuring clear complexion and bodily strength. If there is indigestion, the nutritional essence that nourishes the body will be affected and this will impede the development of the bodily constituents. Therefore, protecting digestive heat with proper diet and lifestyle can ensure good health and longevity.

TABLE 7.1

Diet according to humoral typology

	WIND/*LOONG*	BILE/*TRIPA*	PHLEGM/*BEKEN*
General	Warm, nutritious, oily foods	Fresh, cooling foods	Hot, spicy, and light foods
Drinks	Warm water, herbal teas (chamomile, caraway, fennel, anise, nettle), milk, red wine	Boiled cooled water/ fresh water, green, black tea, beer, fresh fruit juice	Hot water, ginger tea, green tea, black tea, black coffee, small amount of strong alcohol
Vegetables	Radish, onion, garlic, pumpkin, carrots, leeks celery, seaweed, beans, mushrooms, potatoes, eggplant, corn	Broccoli, carrots, cucumbers, zucchini, cabbage, lettuce, bell peppers, chicory, beets, spinach, rucola, tomatoes, peas	Dried or cooked radish, horseradish, broccoli, nettle, pumpkin, seaweed, peppers, rhubarb, tomatoes, spinach, asparagus, leeks, squash
Grains and legumes	Rice, millet, oats, quinoa, lentils, beans, soybeans	Rice, buckwheat, millet, quinoa, lentils	Rice, buckwheat, oats, quinoa, chickpeas, lentils, beans
Meats	Mutton, lamb, beef, duck, chicken, fish, eggs	Goat, fresh beef, fresh pork, herbivorous game (deer, etc.)	Fish, mutton, lamb, pork, beef, duck, chicken, rabbit, hare
Oils	Ghee, 1 year aged butter, sesame oil, linseed oil, cow and sheep butter, marrow	Fresh butter, ghee, olive oil, almond oil, coconut oil	Olive oil, sesame oil, ghee, coconut oil
Dairy	Cow's, sheep's, and goat's milk, yogurt, cooked yogurt, fresh cheese, aged cheese	Skim milk, goat's milk, yogurt, kefir, fresh cheese	Whey (cheese water), cooked yogurt, buttermilk
Spices	Coriander, nutmeg, clove, cardamom, pepper, cumin, mustard, salt	Saffron, clove, turmeric, mint, basil	Chili, pepper, cumin, mustard, ginger, anise, cinnamon, cardamom, salt

People with allergies should avoid the problematic items, even if they are listed in the table. In cases of special medical conditions please consult your physician, whether Western or Tibetan, before making any dietary changes.

TABLE 7.2

Recommended lifestyle according to humoral typology

	WIND/*LOONG*	BILE/*TRIPA*	PHLEGM/*BEKEN*
General	Regular lifestyle, especially regular eating and sleeping times	Regular eating and resting	Regular physical activity
Locations	Warm, cozy places; pleasant smells; music	Cool, shady places	Warm, dry, and bright places
Work	6–7 hours (mental or physical)	7–8 hours (mental or physical)	8–9 hours (preferably physical)
Sports	Soft, noncompetitive sports; yoga, jogging, dancing	Soft, noncompetitive sports; swimming, yoga	Boxing, weight lifting, martial arts, dancing, and other vigorous exercise
Free-time activities	Socializing; spending time in nature or with friends and family, not on social networks	Relaxing, reading, avoiding overworking and stress	Gym, brisk walking, outdoor activities; spending time with friends and family, not on social networks
Home self-therapies	Self massage with oil	Cold compress	Hot bath or salt compress
Colors	Yellow, red	White	Blue, green
Sexual intercourse	Moderate	Moderate	Regular
Sleep	8–9 hours	7–8 hours	6–7 hours
Meditation	Mind-calming meditation, breathing exercises	Insight meditation, analytic meditation, breathing exercises	Mindful walking, prostrations
Exercises from Tibetan healing yoga, *nejang*	Exercises for sense organs, head, and limbs	Exercises for head, trunk, and belly	Exercises for waist and legs
Essentials	Nourishing	Detoxification	Fasting

RELAX, be in warm places in the shade, dedicate some time to pleasant conversations with friends and listen to relaxing music. Avoid places with big lakes or near the ocean, places where animals suffer (slaughterhouses, industrial farms, etc.), and high altitudes.

DIET AND LIFESTYLE RECOMMENDATIONS FOR
BILE/*TRIPA* IMBALANCES

One should consume fresh foods like cottage cheese, fresh butter, tofu, beef, goat, chicken or duck, barley soup, vegetable soup (without oil or salt), turnip greens, dandelion, chicory, artichokes, and all bitter vegetables, with porridges. Drink fresh water, mineral water, tepid water, or boiled water that has cooled, goat's or cow's yogurt, goat's milk, and buttermilk.

Live in a cool and softly ventilated area, simplify your life to avoid frenetic energy and triggers to anger, and generally reduce stress as much as possible.

DIET AND LIFESTYLE RECOMMENDATIONS FOR
PHLEGM/*BEKEN* DISORDERS

One should consume warm foods; eat mutton, deer, or wild meat, fish, legumes, and dehydrated vegetables or those that have a dry quality. Drink hot water, especially before meals, yogurt, buttermilk, whey, red wine, or drinks with high alcoholic content.

Live in warm and bright places, dress in comfortable and warm clothes, and commit to regular physical activity such as walking, prostrations, or sports.

Nejang—Tibetan Healing Yoga

Tibetan yoga, known as *tsaloong trulkhor*, is divided into two main parts: the preliminaries and the actual practice. The preliminary part is called *lujong*, meaning body training or body exercise. These body exercises help to balance internal energies, open the channels, and relax the mind. One division of lujong is called *nejang*, meaning cleaning the energy sites in the body. This is used especially to rebalance internal energies for healing. The practice was transmitted by Puton Rinchen Drub (1290–1364) in his Kalachakra[3] teaching system. Nejang is also typically used by Tibetan physicians and is a recommended exercise for patients.

---

[3] Sanskrit: Kālacakra, Tibetan: *dus kyi 'khor lo*; means wheel of time or time cycles. The Kalachakra tradition is a very complex teaching and practice in Tibetan Buddhism, revolving around the concept of time (*kāla*) and cycles (*chakra*), from the cycles of the planets to the cycles of human breathing. It teaches the practice of working with the most subtle energies within the body on the path to enlightenment.

Nejang is a combination of breathing, movements, and self massage. There are twenty-four movements. Here I will explain some basic ones that are beneficial for imbalances according to the three humors. The healing benefits of the exercises are given according to both the tantric text as well as medical tradition. Before beginning nejang, it is recommended to do the ninefold purification breathing. To begin nejang, first sit with a straight back; inhale and hold the breath, compressing the energy in the navel; do the movements/massage; then exhale superficially, like shooting an arrow from your nose. Repeat each exercise at least three times or for five to ten minutes.

Nejang for Wind/Loong Imbalances

EAR EXERCISE

This exercise pacifies the wind in the muscles and the complexion. It also balances the kidneys, gives stability to the spine, and strengthens the urinary bladder and reproductive organs.

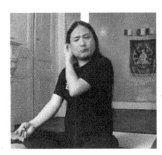 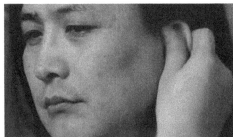

Method: Inhale, hold the breath in the belly, and begin to massage the right ear with your left hand. Massage the ear from top to bottom, pressing intermittently on pain points or areas that feel hard. Repeat as many times as possible while holding the breath. Then exhale through the nose superficially, i.e., do not fully empty or collapse the belly. Repeat at least three times, then do the same for the left ear with the right hand.

TONGUE EXERCISE

According to the tantric text, this exercise is good for brain disorders, and according to medical tradition, it is for disorders of the heart and small intestine, and emotional blockages such as sadness, depression, and lack of memory. It is a simple but profound exercise to balance the wind/*loong* humor.

Method: Inhale, hold the breath in the belly, and begin to stretch the

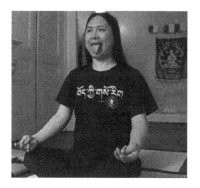

tongue in four directions, up, down, right, left; then fully stretch out the tongue and rotate it three times clockwise and counterclockwise. Repeat the exercise at least three times.

CROWN POINT MASSAGE

This exercise helps stiffness of limbs, especially difficulty in extension and contraction. It pacifies all winds, calms the mind, and treats the mind as well as overthinking. It also helps breathing and stimulates brain circulation.

Method: First, warm the palms by rubbing the hands together briskly.

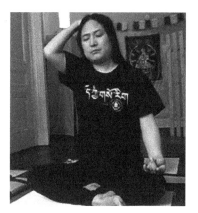

Then place the warm palm of your hand over the crown of the head. Repeat a few times. To begin the massage, inhale, hold the breath by compressing the energy in the navel, then rub the crown of the head strongly with the palm. Then rest your hands and exhale superficially. Repeat at least three times.

Nejang for Bile/Tripa Imbalances

EYE EXERCISE

As the eyes are the flower with the root in the liver, it will come as no surprise that exercising the eyes will strengthen the liver. This exercise not

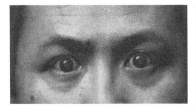 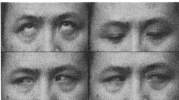

only heals the eyes but also balances the liver, gall bladder, pancreas, and bile humor.

Method: Just as we need to stretch our muscles before exercising, we try to stretch the muscles of our eyes before moving them in four directions. Inhale, hold the breath, and open the eyes as wide as possible. Then gaze in the four directions and make a full rotation clockwise and counterclockwise while fully stretching the eye muscles. Exhale superficially. Repeat at least three times.

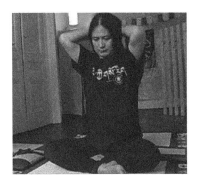

NECK MASSAGE

Besides eye problems, other common issues caused by bile/*tripa* imbalances are manifestations of tension and pain in the upper part of the body, tendency to baldness, and frequent headaches.

This exercise can help to stop hair loss and strengthen the eyes, kidneys, and spleen. It is also helpful for headaches, relaxing the neck, and releasing tension.

Method: Inhale, hold the breath, clasp the hands, and strongly massage the back of the head and occipital region. Massage by rubbing and squeezing with clasped hands for as long as possible while holding the breath. Then release the hands and exhale superficially. Repeat at least three times, i.e., three breaths.

THIGH MASSAGE

According to the tantric text, this exercise helps to pacify blood problems. And according to the medical tradition, it pacifies hot-natured diseases

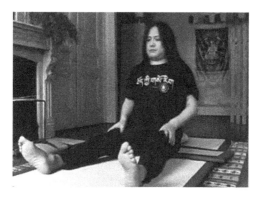

(inflammation, infection, fever), balances bile/*tripa*, stimulates circulation, strengthens the immune system, and protects the body.

Method: Inhale, hold the breath, and strongly massage the thighs by rubbing, kneading, and hitting. Massage for as long as you can hold your breath, then exhale superficially. Repeat at least three times.

Nejang for Phlegm/Beken *Imbalances*

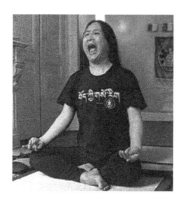

LIP EXERCISE

This exercise is good for stomach problems, the spleen, and abdominal pain.

Method: Inhale, hold the breath, tightly purse the lips together, then stretch open the mouth as wide as possible. Exhale and repeat at least three times.

ROTATING THE BELLY EXERCISE

Typical problems of phlegm/*beken* imbalance are slow digestion and a feeling of internal cold. This very important exercise helps to improve digestion, unblock constipation, and build up body energy. It is also helpful for problems in the legs and stomach.

Method: Inhale deeply and visualize filling up a round vase that is located in the navel with your breath. Hold the breath, compressing the energy in the navel by gently contracting the anal sphincter, and begin to rotate the belly clockwise for a minimum of three rounds and counterclockwise for a minimum of three rounds. Then draw the abdomen in and out for a minimum of three times while still holding the breath. Then exhale superficially, like shooting an arrow from your nose, 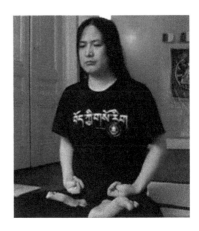 and repeat the exercise. As your breathing capacity increases, it will be beneficial to gradually increase the number of rotations (clockwise and counterclockwise) and numbers of in/out belly movements in each breath to make seven, fourteen, or twenty-one rounds. You can do this whole exercise for twenty-one sets or from ten to twenty minutes.

ANKLE MASSAGE

This exercise helps to cure backaches and pains. It also helps the kidneys and balances menstruation.

Method: Inhale, hold the breath, and strongly rub and massage both ankles. Exhale and repeat at least three times.

It is recommended to end the ne-jang session with silent relaxation or meditation. A simple way is to allow the body and mind to rest by simply observing the breath.

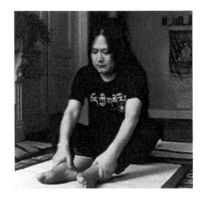

The Seasons and How They Affect the Three Humors

In Sowa Rigpa there are two ways to view the seasons. One way involves the traditional four seasons, with an intermediate "season" in between one season and the next. The other is the traditional subdivision of the year into six parts. According to the external elements and how they affect the body, care should be taken to prevent strain on the affected organs. With the knowledge of your typology, extra care and steps can be taken in each season to maintain humoral balance.

The Seasons and the Five External Elements

The universal energies of nature manifest cyclically with the seasons' elemental energies emerging from the earth, progressively increasing in intensity until the energy peaks and is then reabsorbed back into the earth, manifesting the intermediate season (the transitional time between one season and the next). Each season has characteristics according to the predominant astrological element. In spring one should have a light diet so as not to overload the liver; purify the liver by drinking saffron water; and be careful not to overstress oneself with physical activity.

In summer, one should focus on the heart from both a physiological and an emotional point of view. One should get adequate physical activity. During this season, it is helpful to use nutmeg.

In autumn we can help the lungs by using bamboo pith or gentian. One should also avoid dairy because it increases phlegm. During the autumn, it is important to do intense physical activity.

In winter, the kidneys are helped by consuming green cardamom and continuing the activity level of the autumn.

During the intermediate seasons, the spleen and stomach benefit from the use of black cardamom and pomegranate fruit or powder respectively.

Generally, consume fruit and greens that are available in each season, as they have the vital energy to balance the season and help maintain health.

The Seasons and the Five Internal Elements

Another traditional understanding of the seasons divides the year into six parts. The year is first divided at the two solstices; then each part is further divided into three phases. Each phase is associated with an elemental

TABLE 7.3

Seasons, elements, and tastes

WINTER SOLSTICE, DECEMBER 21

Season	End of winter	Spring	End of spring
Elements	Fire-wind	Earth-wind	Water-wind
Tastes	Spicy	Astringent	Bitter

SUMMER SOLSTICE, JUNE 21

Season	Summer	Autumn	Winter
Elements	Fire-earth	Water-fire	Earth-water
Tastes	Sour	Salty	Sweet

combination and one of the six tastes. It is important not to use the five external elements and the five internal elements in the same analysis. They represent two different energetic levels. The external elements are the most common method for addressing health and are simpler to balance. The five internal elements are much deeper and represent more subtle aspects; therefore, more spiritual training is required to work at that level.

Traditionally, one begins with the period following the winter solstice. The first period is the transition from the end of winter into spring. This season has the elemental combination of fire and wind and a spicy taste. Starting with the winter solstice, there is the end-of-winter transition, spring, spring transition, the summer solstice, autumn, and the beginning of winter.

Each season is associated with elemental combinations that produce its characteristic taste.

Every plant has a biological clock that relates to the seasons and determines its nature. As the plant grows in each season, the characteristic flavor of the season infuses it and gives the practitioner a clue to its medicinal properties.

The period from the beginning until the end of winter is characterized by a very strong energy in the body. In fact, the body dissipates less metabolic heat and produces energy to resist the cold. In spring and autumn the energetic level is medium. At the end of spring and in summer it is weaker, as from the moment the seasonal temperature rises, the internal metabolism dissipates.

These energy fluctuations are connected with accumulation, manifestation, and pacification of the humors in the body during particular seasons.

Accumulation, Manifestation, and Pacification of the Three Humors

In a particular season, each energy either accumulates, manifests, or is pacified. Accumulation, manifestation, and pacification have their causes: nature and their time. The three energies do not become imbalanced suddenly as disorders go through stages of development. At first the environmental factors lead to an accumulation or increase in the humoral energy. Then incorrect diet or behavioral patterns can lead to a manifestation. Manifestation happens when a cause (seasons, diet, or lifestyle) is accumulated excessively. In pacification, the body rebalances the accumulation or increase in humoral energy and balance is restored.

The wind/*loong* energy accumulates at the end of spring, manifests in summer, and is pacified in autumn. The energy of bile/*tripa* accumulates in the summer, explodes in autumn, and is pacified in winter. Phlegm/*beken* accumulates in winter, manifests in spring, and is pacified at the end of spring.

The energies, whether wind/*loong*, bile/*tripa*, or phlegm/*beken*, are always present in our body in all seasons, not just during the periods in which they accumulate, manifest, or are pacified.

During all stages of accumulation (end of spring, summer, and winter), it is particularly important to apply diet, herbs, and spices to pacify the appropriate humor and prevent the possible emergence of disorders. If, however, you are not able to prevent the accumulation of the humor, use substances that help in its elimination.

Spring

In spring, to maintain balance during the manifestation of phlegm/ *beken*, we should drink ginger tea, or simply hot water. It is advisable to eat little red meat and to consume fish, sweetened with honey if necessary. If excessive *beken* manifests, emetic substances should be administered to

TABLE 7.4

The three humors during the seasons

SEASONS	WIND/*LOONG*	BILE/*TRIPA*	PHLEGM/*BEKEN*
Beginning and end of winter (November to February)	Normal state	Pacification	Accumulation
Beginning of spring (March and April)	Normal state	Normal state	Manifestation
End of spring (May and June)	Accumulation	Normal state	Pacification
Summer (July and August)	Manifestation	Accumulation	Normal state
Autumn (September and October)	Pacification	Manifestation	Normal state

induce vomiting.[4] To reduce the accumulation of wind/*loong*, it is appropriate to drink clove tea and eat regularly, using spicy foods and fruits.

Summer

In summer, with the high external temperature, skin pores dilate, causing a dispersion of internal body heat, which in turn causes depletion of physical energy. Due to the loss of metabolic heat that slows down digestion, we should take light food. Therefore, avoid or at least reduce cold drinks and any kind of cold food and also cut down on the consumption of dairy products. Less aggressive methods like steaming or boiling are preferred in food preparation. It is advisable to eat cooked and tepid food that restores the metabolic body heat and the energy. Consume food enriched by the use of saffron and turmeric to avoid the excessive accumulation of bile/*tripa*, typical in this period. Consuming fruits and vegetables of the season facilitates the hydrous balance. In case of excessive wind/*loong* manifestation, laxatives should be administered.

---

[4] According to the tree of therapy—the fourth trunk of external therapies—for cleansing; emetics are best for excessive phlegm, purgative methods are best for excessive bile, and enemas best for excessive wind.

Autumn

In autumn, the period in which bile/*tripa* manifests, it is preferable to consume light foods, raw, fresh, or undercooked. Avoid dairy and fatty foods that are difficult to digest. Instead of alcohol, drink saffron tisanes. With these food solutions, a balanced humor manifestation is favored. Otherwise, purgative substances are administrated to limit an excessive manifestation of *tripa*.

Winter

In winter, when phlegm/*beken* accumulates, it is indicated to eat cooked hot food and avoid dishes that are very heavy and elaborate. Limit the intake of milk and dairy products and use grains and their derivatives moderately. The consumption of wine, particularly red, which possesses the characteristics to rebalance *beken*, is recommended. Decoctions and tisanes of ginger are also indicated, and drinking hot water before eating.

In winter, with the severe cold, the pores close, which results in stronger inner heat and body strength. We must still eat nutritious foods, fats, and oils, as there is an increased demand for energy, but not too much. It is a great practice to receive massages to warm up. The body, properly nurtured and heated, is reinforced due to strong metabolic heat.

Nature of Hot and Cold Foods

To understand which foods are adequate for a certain humor, we categorize them based on their cold or hot nature.

The nature of a particular food is determined by the environment in which it grows, or by its properties. Plants in dry locations have the fire nature, which is hot. To this group belong cereals, some fruits, vegetables, spices, and honey. However, onions and garlic growing under the earth possess hot and spicy nature.

The foods that thrive in a land that has a lot of water or have a high percentage of fat are of cold nature. In this category are the roots, greens, fish, mollusks, seaweeds, milk, yogurt, and coconut.

Cooking methods and the processes of preparation modify foods' properties. Boiling, steaming, frying, and baking can change the texture and taste of food, thereby changing its therapeutic properties. Here, again we have to consider the five elements. For example, boiling introduces the element of water, which has the nature of smoothness and fluidity, into the food; therefore it would help to pacify wind/*loong* and bile/*tripa*. Baking uses dry heat and therefore is good for counteracting the stickiness and coldness in phlegm/*beken*. However, in general, heating food makes it more digestible and promotes digestive heat.

The hot foods stimulate the digestive heat, while the cold ones tend to weaken the digestion.

When the humors are in balance, it is advisable to eat tepid foods, to avoid stimulating the three energies excessively.

Cold and raw foods can cool the interior of the body. And if such a diet is maintained for a long time, it can cause weak digestive heat and the arousal of pathologies.

Taste in Relation to Hot and Cold

Another important aspect of foods is their flavor, a quality that is perceived by the tongue. Due to particular reflexes of the mouth, we can affirm that the sweet taste adheres to the tongue. The sour taste adheres to the teeth and causes abundant salivation. The salty taste generates heat and increases salivation, the bitter eliminates halitosis and humidifies the mouth, and finally, the astringent adheres to the palate, giving a feeling of roughness.

Spicy foods like pepper, paprika, and ginger; sour foods like lemon and citrus in general; vinegar, wine, and other alcoholic products; all products that have gone through fermentation; and salty foods belong to the category of hot flavors.

The cold flavors are bitter, astringent, and sweet.

The bitter flavor substances are used as antipyretics to cool the body or to cleanse. They are mainly used for afflictions caused by bile imbalances or for liver changes because of their ability to reduce liver heat.

It is important to remember that:

- The hot substances increase bile/*tripa* and lessen wind/*loong* and phlegm/*beken*.

TABLE 7.5

Relationships among tastes, kind of energy to which they belong, elements from which they are formed, and relationships with the three humors

TASTES	ENERGY	ELEMENTS	INCREASING	PACIFICATION
Sour	Hot	Fire-earth	Bile/*tripa*	Wind/*loong*—phlegm/*beken*
Bitter	Cold	Water-air	Wind/*loong*—phlegm/*beken*	Bile/*tripa*
Astringent	Cold	Earth-air	Wind/*loong*—phlegm/*beken*	Bile/*tripa*
Sweet	Cold	Earth-water	Phlegm/*beken*	Wind/*loong*—bile/*tripa*
Spicy	Hot	Fire-air	Bile/*tripa*	Phlegm/*beken*
Salty	Hot	Fire-water	Bile/*tripa*	Wind/*loong*—phlegm/*beken*

- Cold substances purify and calm bile/*tripa* as well as stimulate, tone, and tighten the tissues.
- The spicy increases bile/*tripa* and pacifies phlegm/*beken*.
- The sour increases bile/*tripa* and pacifies wind/*loong* and phlegm/*beken*.
- The bitter and astringent increases wind/*loong* and phlegm/*beken* and pacifies bile/*tripa*.
- The sweet increases phlegm/*beken* and pacifies wind/*loong* and bile/*tripa*.
- The salty increases wind/*loong* and phlegm/*beken* and pacifies bile/*tripa*.

To understand how the effects of food change if they are hot or cold and which is the predominant taste, it is useful to try them ourselves and observe the reaction that they cause.

Herbal Medicines

The use of herbal substances is one of the main healing methods of Sowa Rigpa, along with diet, lifestyle, and external therapies. The pharmacology dates back to ancient times and consists largely of medicinal plants found on the high plateau and in the mountainous regions of Tibet. Unlike modern Western medications, which are made from isolated chemical compounds, Sowa Rigpa formulas are compounded from a variety of different natural substances, predominantly of plant origin, as well as some minerals.

Fundamental to medicinal compounding in Sowa Rigpa is the theory of interdependent function, wherein the characteristics of the external five elements are utilized therapeutically within multicomponent formulae to cure imbalances of the five elements that involve the physical body in a more subtle form. These multicomponent medicinal formulae have profound effects in curing systemic disorders, as they not only target the main organ specifically but also support the entire organ system, as well as allied organs, tissues, and energetic pathways.

In essence, Sowa Rigpa medicinal formulae can be divided into two broad categories: medicines that have a warm nature and those that have a cool nature. Hot- or warm-natured medicines are used to cure cold conditions; cold- or cool-natured medicines are used to cure disorders of heat.

According to Sowa Rigpa, all medicinal substances, including food substances, have different innate powers or potencies that can cure dysfunction due to imbalance of the energies of the body. There are considered to be eight predominant powers or potencies:

Heavy
Light
Hot
Cool
Blunt
Sharp
Coarse
Oily

In addition, all the substances contain particular tastes. This is very important, as each taste has a special power to cure imbalances of the three humors. Just as the taste of food is used to balance the humors, Tibetan medications can be classified according to taste and potency.

Medications for imbalance of wind/*loong* according to taste and potency:

Taste: sweet, sour, salty
Potency: oily, heavy, smooth

Medications for imbalance of bile/*tripa* according to taste and potency:

Taste: sweet, bitter, astringent
Potency: cool, subtle, blunt

Medications for imbalance of phlegm/*beken* according to taste and potency:

Taste: pungent, sour, astringent
Potency: sharp, rough, light

In a few cases, single herbs are used for curing specific single non-complex disorders, although this is the exception to the rule, taking into account the complexity of the human organism. Spices, condiments, and foods can be use as therapeutic substances when their properties are known and if administered in a timely manner and method.

The general indications to consider are:

Substances that are beneficial for wind/*loong* diseases should contain sweet (sugarcane), sour (wine, vinegar, pomegranate), and salty (red salt or Himalayan salt) tastes and have the qualities of viscosity (bark aquilaria extract), heaviness (black salt), and softness (chamomile).

The substances that help in bile/*tripa* disorders should have sweet (raisins), bitter (bitter cucumber), and astringent (white sandalwood) tastes and contain the cold (camphor), liquid (cassia shells), and calming (bamboo culm) qualities.

The substances to treat phlegm/*beken* imbalances should have hot (black pepper), bitter or sour (pomegranate), and astringent (*Terminalia belerica*) tastes and sharp (salt), rough (bramble), and light (ginger) qualities.

The medicinal effects of the pharmacopeia can be used to limit or eliminate disorders. Prescribing substances or formulas based on tastes pacifies and calms the excess humor. Using substances or formulas based on qualities eliminates the disorder.

To pacify malnutrition caused by wind/*loong*, one should prescribe medicines such as meat broth, "broth with the four essences" (meat, wine, sugarcane, and butter), medicated butter with nutmeg or garlic, the three fruits of the myrobalan,[5] or the five roots.[6] To eliminate wind/*loong*, one should prescribe daily enemas that can be light, medium, or strong.

To calm bile/*tripa* disorders, one can use chebulic myrobalan decoctions, elecampane, or a decoction of the three fruits. One can also use powders of camphor, white sandalwood, saffron, bamboo pith, or kaolin.

To calm the phlegm/*beken* imbalances, one uses medicinal pills that contain ginger, black aconite, or a mixture of salts (e.g., table salt, Himalayan rock salt, and black salt), as well as the ashes of burnt pomegranate, rhododendron, black pepper, or calcite.

Please refer to appendix 1 for a list of herbs, foods, and spices used in Sowa Rigpa for healing.

---

[5] The three fruits: cherubic myrobalan (*Terminalia chebula Retz.*), belliric myrobalan (*Terminalia bellirica Roxb.*), and gooseberry (*Emblica officinalis Gaertn* [Syn. *phyllanthus emblica Linn*]).

[6] The five roots: pleurospermum (*pleurospermum tibetanicum Wolff*), Solomon's seal (*polygonatum verticillatum L.*), asparagus (*asparagus adscendens Roxb.*), caltrop (*tribulus terrestris Linn.* [Syn. *T. Lanuguinosus L.*]), winter cherry (*withania somnifera*).

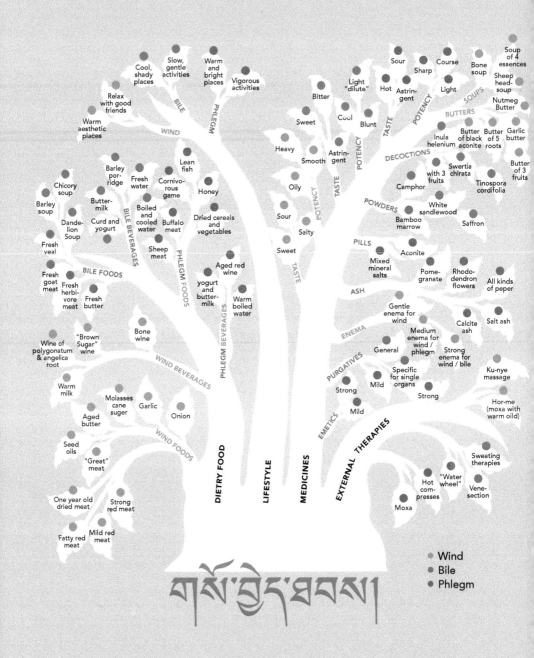

FIG. 21. The Tree of Therapies Highlighting the Trunk of External Therapies

8

External Therapies

In Sowa Rigpa, external therapies are an integral part of healing. They play a fundamental role, as different treatments are applied in specific ways according to the problem.

Massage therapy, known as *kunye*, can be easily applied in a variety of ways to treat most diseases. Together with Mongolian moxa (*horme*), *kunye* remains the foremost treatment for wind/*loong* pathologies.

Hot baths, sauna, and hydrotherapy or water wheel (cold water sprayed on affected areas) are indicated for bile/*tripa* diseases because these therapies induce perspiration. Bloodletting is also used for this kind of imbalance.

Hot compresses, poultices, and the use of moxa are preferred for phlegm/*beken* imbalances.

Chapter Outline

TRUNK OF EXTERNAL THERAPIES (3 BRANCHES)

I. Branch of wind/*loong* (2 leaves)
    A. *Kunye*

B. *Horme*
II. Branch of bile/*tripa* (3 leaves)
  A. Bloodletting
  B. Sweating therapies
  C. Cold water therapies
III. Branch of phlegm/*beken* (2 leaves)
  A. Moxa
  B. Hot compresses

Kunye Massage

Kunye originated in the ancient Tibetan kingdom more than 3,900 years ago and is a native practice of the Tibetan medical tradition. Formerly, Tibetans used *kunye* for diagnosis and to treat imbalances of constitution with applications of oil infusions. Tree branches, sticks, and stones were widely used as part of the therapy, to exert pressure on different parts and points of the body with the aim of restoring the health and well-being of the individual.

The full name of Tibetan massage is *ku nye chi*. The Tibetan word illustrates the three phases of the massage: *ku* = oil application; *nye* = massage; *chi* = oil removal. Literally, *ku* means "apply," or to anoint the body with therapeutic oils that are absorbed through the skin, and *nye* refers to the massage itself. The *nye* technique includes stroking, kneading, rubbing, and applying pressure on the muscles and tendons, as well as on several points and channels. *Chi*, the final part of *kunye*, involves cleaning the oils off the body using barley or chickpea powder. Other ingredients can be added to the powder base, depending on the condition and the diagnosis of the person. Another common name for *kunye* is *chugpa* (Tib. *byugpa*).

Kunye belongs to the fourth category of treatment, external therapies, after diet, lifestyle, and medicine. It is part of the valuable external therapies of traditional Tibetan medicine, used to heal or restore balance. The rejuvenating benefits and restorative function of *kunye* are mentioned in many original Tibetan texts, including *Bum Shi, Gyu Shi* and all of its medical commentaries, and the medical text *Ton Huang*. The benefits include the elimination of toxins that accumulate in the body, increased vitality, and reduction and alleviation of several kinds of pain.

In modern society, nobody is free from stress connected to work and psychological pressures. Massage can be an excellent therapy for wind/

loong disorders arising from these disturbances. Therefore, it is advisable for both sick people and those in good health.

Now, let's have a closer look at the particular phases of *kunye*.

The *ku* massage is divided into three main parts: oil application (Tib. *chugpa*); joint mobilization (Tib. *tsig jor*); and heat application (Tib. *sowa*). The oil used is specific according to the patient's typology. Sesame oil with nutmeg, cloves, and aniseed is used if working with wind/*loong*; olive oil with saffron for bile/*tripa* typology; and sunflower seed oil or sesame with ginger if the person is mostly phlegm/*beken*. Before the oil application, it is necessary to heat the massage oil so that absorption through the skin is facilitated and helps to relax the body and calm the mind through the substances contained in the oil. The body of the patient is divided into three parts; the right side is where the bile/*tripa* energy is predominant, the central part is dominated by wind/*loong*, and the left side by phlegm/*beken*. The central part is oiled first, followed by the sides, with care not to heat the right part too much, because the bile/*tripa* energy is already a hot energy. The oil should be distributed all over the body and should also be fully absorbed into the skin to enhance blood and energetic circulation.

Together with increased blood circulation, we perform mobilization of the joints and the centers of the minor chakras (*khorlo*, literally "wheel"), so as to reactivate the energetic circulation in places where it has stagnated. Besides that, because each part and limb of the body has a relationship with an internal organ, the mobilization also acts on those organs.

Before massaging a person in good health, it is very important to know their type of humoral constitution. Each typology requires the application of specific oils and herbs on different points of the body.

Tibetan medicine subdivides the life of an individual into several phases, which are associated with the three humors in the following way:

Early childhood (under 2): phlegm/*beken*
Childhood (age 2 to 16): wind/*loong*
Maturity/adulthood (age 16 to 70): bile/*tripa*
Old age (over 70): wind/*loong*

Kunye massage is particularly indicated for children and teenagers less than 16 years old and for the elderly who are more than 70 years old, the ages in which the humor wind/*loong* is predominant.

The hot or cold application is done according to the typology of the patient. For wind/*loong* and phlegm/*beken* types, warm compresses with stones or salt are used to warm up cold areas; for bile/*tripa* types, cold compresses with cold stones or crystals are used on hot points.

Oil Application

Different quantities and types of oil are to be used according to the different typologies. If the dominant humor of the patient is wind/*loong*, his skin is dry and his body is colder. More oil should be applied and the massage should be vigorous. If the patient has a phlegm/*beken* constitution, less oil is applied, so the friction will be stronger. If the body is very hot (bile/*tripa* typology), saffron or turmeric decoctions are applied instead of oil.

Some Tibetan doctors only perform *ku* massage with several oils, while others specialize in *nye* massage without oil. *Lon nye* means wet massage, done with oils. *Kam nye* means dry massage, done without the use of oils.

THE OILS FOR MASSAGE

These are just some examples of commonly used herbs and oils.

  Oils for wind/*loong* typology: sesame oil with aniseed, nutmeg, and cloves
  Oils for bile/*tripa* typology: sandalwood oil, extra virgin olive oil, or almond oil; a bit of saffron is added to one liter of oil, which is left to infuse for a week in the shade and exposed overnight in the moonlight. Instead of saffron, which is very expensive, dried calendula flowers can be used. The oil prepared in this manner will have refreshing characteristics.
  Oils for phlegm/*beken* typology: sesame or sunflower oil with ginger and coriander

The chakra of heat, i.e., the palms of the hands, is used to apply the oil.

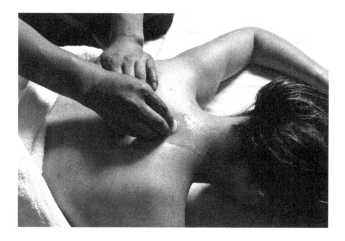

FIG. 22. Oil application

MASSAGE INSTRUCTIONS

First, check the temperature of your hands. If they are cold, rub them together until they are warm. This will facilitate the oil absorption. Next, look for the coldest part of the patient's body and warm it. If the whole body is cold, it has to be rubbed and hit lightly to warm up. You can also warm up one part at a time, from head to shoulders, shoulders to navel, etc. If possible, women's breasts should also be warmed. During the massage the parts that are not being treated should be kept warm.

The head is very important, because it is the center of wind/*loong*. The *loong* descends from the head to the rest of the body through the channels; therefore the oil application starts from the head.

The right side of the body is massaged softly, since this part is usually hotter, being connected to bile/*tripa* fire.

The left side of the body is massaged more strongly and vigorously, since it is colder, connected with the cold energy of phlegm/*beken*.

When the massage with oil application is done well, the patient's cheeks can appear flushed. This is a good sign that the regenerative energy has been activated and the massage has reached the constituent factors of the body. This energy showing up in the cheeks is intimately related to the heart energy, which regulates the face color.

Joint Mobilization

In Sowa Rigpa, the joints are considered the centers of the minor chakras, the true body's energy centers. We balance the various minor chakras located in the joints with movements and the energy of fire represented by the therapist's palm. Applying the principles of Sowa Rigpa to balance hot with cold and vice versa, for example, putting the palm, center of the fire chakra, on the elbow, the center of the wind chakra, will rebalance the cold air with heat. Apply heat to the soles of the feet, the center of the chakra of blood, because without heat, blood cannot circulate. Since blood is liquid, it contains the energy of phlegm/*beken*, which is cold, but also the hot energy of bile/*tripa*, the body's motor. Giving warmth to the blood improves circulation.

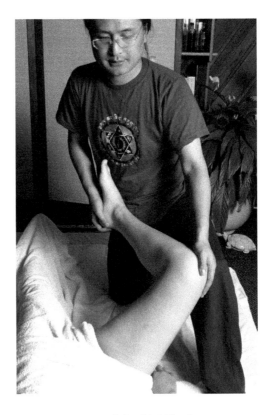

FIG. 23. Joint Mobilization

TABLE 8.1
Relationships between joints and chakras

ARTICULATION	CHAKRA ELEMENT	NATURE
Right palm	Fire	Hot
Left palm	Earth	Cold
Elbows	Air	Neutral
Knees	Water	Cold
Soles of feet	Blood	Hot/cold

Treating the joints, the therapist works and connects the different chakras/*khorlo* to harmonize them.

The wind chakra, *loong khorlo* (neutral), is located at the elbow. Even if it is neutral during the massage, it tends to accentuate the cold potential of this chakra.

The fire chakra, *me khorlo* (heat), is located on the right palm.

The water chakra, *chu khorlo* (cold), is located in the knees.

The earth chakra, *sa khorlo* (cold), is located on the left palm.

The blood chakra, *träg khorlo* (heat), is located on the soles of the feet.

The left palm is considered the center of the earth chakra, but during *kunye* massage, therapist uses both palms as chakras of fire through movement and friction, creating heat. The left palm of the patient corresponds to the earth chakra and the right palm corresponds to the fire chakra.

It is useful to remember that hot energy matches bile/*tripa*, cold energy matches phlegm/*beken*, and neutral energy matches wind/*loong*.

Mobilizations are performed on the major joints of the body: shoulders, elbows, wrists, hips, knees, and ankles, and on some smaller joints like those in the fingers and toes. The head and legs are treated when the patient lies on his back. It is important to warm up each part (elbows, knees, etc.), with the palms first.

Through mobilization and massage, we can remove the excess of all-pervasive wind and connective phlegm that stays in the joints and may limit motion.

In Sowa Rigpa, each limb is connected to a full organ. As a result, working on the limbs and on the joints has a direct effect on the health of the organs to which they are connected.

TABLE 8.2

Relationships between limbs and solid organs

LIMB	SOLID ORGAN
Left arm	Spleen
Left leg	Kidneys
Right arm	Liver
Right leg	Lungs
Head	Heart

HEAT APPLICATION

After the application of oil and mobilization of joints, parts of the body must be heated to facilitate the absorption of oil and the therapeutic substances contained within through the pores. This amplifies the effects of massage and relaxation.

The best method of heat application is wrapping heated stones in towels and placing them on different areas of the body, based on the patient's

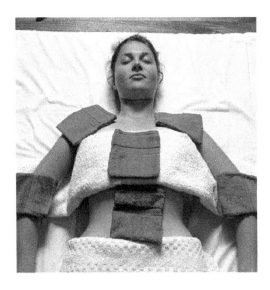

FIG. 24. Heating the *beken* locations

typology. Alternatively, the therapist can rub their hands together briskly to create heat and place them on specific areas.

In summer, the patient may lie in the sun; in winter, they should be near a fireplace or a brazier. A natural heat source (rather than an electric heater) should be employed if possible, to avoid interference in the flow of energy.

First warm your hands and then the patient's body—joints, upper stomach, kidneys, ears, eyes, etc.—for two or three minutes. The heating follows the location of three humors: wind/*loong*, bile/*tripa*, and phlegm/*beken*. If the patient's predominant energy is phlegm/*beken*, warm up the knees first, then elbows, kidneys, and stomach. If bile/*tripa* is predominant, heating is not necessary unless some parts such as stomach and kidneys are cold.

Nye—Muscular Massage

Nye, the second part of *ku-nye-chi*, includes the treatment of target points using finger pressure. It is performed with precise maneuvers described below:

Rubbing (*phuri-nye*): heating up certain areas of the body such as meridians, tendons, ligaments, joints, and along the spine

Pressure (*non-nye*): running pressure on muscles, points, and meridians to eliminate stagnant energy and facilitate the entry of dynamic vital energy

Dragging (*ded-nye*): sliding movements with thumbs, palms of the hands, knuckles, and fists

Pinching (*tsir-nye*): done briskly with two fingers

Pulling (*nye-zin*): a lifting movement done by grabbing and strongly lifting the limb muscles

Beating (*nye-deg*): tapping motions on specific points using the fingers

Drumming up (*dung-nye*): fists are used to work on the muscles with different intensity

Point pressure (*sang-nye*): executed at specific points, usually specific moxa, bloodletting, stick therapy, and acupuncture points

Circular pressure (*kor-nye*): on the muscles or on specific areas, with the palm or with the thumbs in a circular or spiraling motion, with gradually increasing strength

Kneading (*tzi-nye*): on the muscles, just like working with dough

Vibrational shaking (*trug-nye*): an open hand on the back and on the limbs

Elongation (*then-nye*): stretching done with the palms, thumbs, wrists or forearms, as though to separate two areas (for example, spine and muscles) between them

Fast rubbing (*drug-nye*): technique performed with both thumbs on bloodletting points to allow heat dispersion

Five-finger technique (*sor-nye*): a series of movement using open fingers on the muscles that includes tapping, shaking, and pinching

In *nye* there are five parts to be massaged: muscles, tendons, energetic points, meridians through which the wind/*loong* energy flows, and skin.

There are many different kinds of muscles, each with a different function. The muscle is treated at three different levels; superficial, intermediate, and deep.

Nye massage involves 45 principal muscles or muscle groups. It relaxes the contracted muscles, brings the energies into balance, and improves muscle function. All muscles are related to each other, so treating thedr principal muscles will benefit all the minor muscles.

Tibetans refer to muscles as white or black/red. White muscles are those connected with wind/*loong* energy (cold) and most of them are tendons, whereas black/red muscles are those connected to solar energy (hot). Rubbing and sliding techniques are used for tendons and more

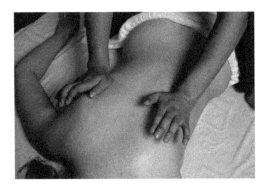

FIG. 25. *Kunye* back massage

kneading, stretching, and pressing for muscles. *Kunye* massage is a method for prevention of muscle damage. The damage or permanent contraction of one or more of these principal muscles interferes with the natural balance of the whole body.

Visceral Massage—Detoxification of Internal Organs

Visceral massage is used in *kunye* massage to stimulate detoxification of the internal organs. Put one hand on top of the other and draw circles on the area corresponding to each organ. Start with wide circular movements and then make the movements gradually smaller, first clockwise and then counterclockwise. The massage must be superficial if the patient cannot stand the pressure. The stomach is the last organ to be treated. Repeat the massage of each organ at least six times.

Now treat the abdominal muscles. If the patient is constipated, try to relax the muscles with outward waving motions to help the peristalsis. In case of dysentery, relieve the pain by placing your warm palms over the area and then grasping and lifting the abdominal muscles.

As explained in chapter 3, each of the five internal elements (space, wind, fire, water, and earth) creates a solid organ, a hollow organ, and the body parts (see table 8.3). Therefore, each organ is connected to a corresponding limb. In Sowa Rigpa we massage the appropriate limb to treat disorders in the related organ. During a *kunye* massage, besides us-

TABLE 8.3

Connections of the organs of human body with the members
and elements of nature

BODY PART		SOLID ORGAN	ELEMENT	ELEMENT IN TIBETAN
Head	is connected to	Heart	Space	*Namkha*
Right leg	is connected to	Lungs	Wind	*Loong*
Right arm	is connected to	Liver	Fire	*Me*
Left leg	is connected to	Kidney	Water	*Chu*
Left arm	is connected to	Spleen	Earth	*Sa*

ing visceral massage on the area of the affected organs to release tension, tone, and detoxify the inner organs, the practitioner will spend more time treating those limbs related to the organs with particular disorders.

Chi—the Removal of Oil

Chi (Tib. *phyis*) is the removal of oil that was not absorbed through the skin. The medical term is *dril phyis*, while the more commonly used term is *bye phur*. It is done by spreading and rubbing selected powders blended with suitable spices or herbs on the body. Then, with a cotton cloth or sponge, remove the powder with some pressure throughout the body, first vertically and then horizontally. In bile/*tripa* typology, sandalwood powder or calendula is added to chickpea flour while taking care not to produce too much heat in the process. In the case of phlegm/*beken*, chickpea flour, peas, and carob are used to help in removing fat and reducing weight.

Contraindications for Kunye Massage

Conditions involving inflammation or infection
Recent fractures/no pressure
Varicose veins directly over affected areas
Recent severe sprains or bruises (less than 48 hours after)
Areas of broken skin, burns, abscesses
Recent whiplash injuries
Severe osteoporosis
Spinal problems causing abnormal sensations in the limbs
Malignancies or tumors, should not be pressed
Any undiagnosed severe pain or worsening condition
Recent operations
Numbness
Intoxication
Shock
Insect/snake bite
Allergies, especially to metal, or sensitivity to an oil/cream/essence
Cancer/AIDS
Nerve damage, no pressure

Applications for Specific Conditions

PREGNANCY

From the nineteenth to twenty-fourth weeks (fifth to sixth months), do not lay the patient prone or do vertebral work. Do not work on belly points. From the fifth month, the patient should not lie on the stomach but sit down or lie on their side instead. No tapping anywhere; do not increase heat too much. Do not work on the fourth toe, as a channel there turns the fetus and can be used in labor. Avoid descending wind/*loong* points or points that bring energy down.

CHILDREN

The channels are still being formed in children, so to prevent damage when massaging, do not apply pressure, apply heat with the thumbs by rubbing them together, and massage only at skin level.

PEOPLE CLOSE TO DEATH

In general, *kunye* calms the energy of wind/*loong*. In this particular situation, it is helpful to work on the points of internal and external channels of the crown, then restimulate the crown point (*tsang bug*), which is linked to consciousness. When treating a person near death, remember to avoid deep pressure.

Contraindications to the Use of Oil During Massage

Oil should not be applied to patients who have slow digestion, poor appetite, rheumatism, arthritis, wounds, edema, allergies to metals and allergic skin reactions (for skin problems, apply oil around but not directly on the affected areas), or bile, liver, and gall bladder disorders.

For all these conditions, decoctions and herbs in water or alcohol are used instead of oil. Apply the decoction over the area for five minutes and then wait a bit. Reapply the decoction for another ten minutes and after a subsequent interval, cover the patient up again for a further twenty minutes.

*Areas of the Body to Be Massaged, According to
Humoral Typology*

In *kunye*, the human body can be divided into three main parts, corresponding to the three general areas of the body where the three humors are located:

From head to shoulders—phlegm/*beken*. It resides mainly at the top of the head, which expands to the entire head

From shoulders to navel—bile/*tripa* resides mainly in the liver and gall bladder, which extends across the upper torso

From navel to feet—wind/*loong* resides mainly in the hip area, which extends across the lower torso

People who have wind/*loong* typology should be handled with particular care in the application of oil and heat to the corresponding body parts.

People who have bile/*tripa* typology must be handled with particular care in the application of oil or decoctions to the specific body parts involved.

In phlegm/*beken* typology, the specific areas to massage or press are the points connected to the stomach, spleen, urinary bladder, and kidneys, and the areas in which these organs are situated.

Those with mixed typologies should be massaged on the body parts that correspond to the centers of the prevailing humors, but can also be massaged at the points and the centers of other humors.

Ideal Environment for Kunye Massage

Massage is beneficial for all wind/*loong* imbalances. The ambience relieves the disorders of wind/*loong*: calm, peaceful, pleasant, free from noise, gossip, or other disturbances, and dimly lit. In the presence of strong light, it is advisable to cover the patient's eyes with a dark cloth.

Outdoor or indoor places are both suitable for a massage as long as they are warm and comfortable. A sunny beach is just perfect.

If done indoors, the massage should be performed close to a fireplace or a natural heat source. It is good to have some plants in the room since they absorb negativities that the patient may release during the massage.

After a certain period of time those plants may die because of the amount of negative energies absorbed during treatments. Light incense to purify the air. Play recordings of natural sounds (water, wind, birds, and the five elements) or soft classical music to help the patient relax their body and mind. A quiet and easy talk helps to establish good relations.

The best season for massage is winter, since the weather is colder and the body holds all the heat and good energies. During this season the bile/*tripa* energy located in the stomach is at its height and the closed pores hold the heat in. But in case of excess heat, digestion is too fast, preventing proper absorption of nutritious substances.

Oil application is very important and helps the patient to relax and warm up. During summer the body is already heated and releases excess heat through the pores, which is why cool decoctions are preferred to oils. In spring or autumn, either oils or decoctions can be used.

The best times of the day for a massage are mornings and evenings. During the rest of the day (noon and night) it is recommended to massage with decoctions instead of oils, since they are more efficacious in restoring the balance of energies. Before any massage the patient should have only a light meal. After a heavy meal, wait at least two hours before the treatment.

During the massage Tibetans wear particular accessories called "precious pills" made from mixtures of precious gemstones, metals, minerals, and herbs. Gemstones like turquoise or herbal pouches containing *arura* (*chebulic myrobalan*) are believed to protect the patient and the practitioner from negative energies.

The environment for practicing *kunye* should produce satisfaction and delight to the five senses (in Tib. *Dod*, desire; *Yontan nga*, five qualities = the five qualities of desire that are manifested through the senses):

Olfaction—disperse natural perfumes or burn therapeutic incense such as Agar 15 or 31, which is specific for inhalation, or Mindroling incense.

Vision—keep the environment warm and semidark (the second tantra says "warm and dark"), because light activates wind/*loong*. Plants, colors, thangkas (Buddhist paintings), and stones should be present.

Touch—use sheets, towels, and blankets that are soft and fluffy. Keep the hands in good condition with trimmed nails.

Hearing—the practitioner should talk with a sweet voice and use
relaxing music like healing mantras or nature soundss.

Taste—offer herbal tea, white tea, or other hot beverages.

In the therapy place, it is important to have the water element, which
can be represented by a container of water with an agate or a Japanese
fountain. All these features help to infuse a sense of relaxation in the environment and balance the energy.

Massage with Stones

Among the special techniques of *kunye* are *donye* (massage with stones),
massage with shells, *yukchö* (stick massage), a treatment for rebalancing
the protective *la* energy, and massage to rebalance the chakras.

Donye, massage with stones, originates from the Lhunding school. The
ideal stone for massage should fit in the palm and thus should be chosen
according to the hand size of the practitioner. Hot stones or cold stones
can be used. Mineral stones like turquoise, agate, quartz, rose quartz, and
hematite are used cold, while stones from streams, rivers, lakes, or the sea
are best for heating, as they usually are not rough or sharp but rounded,
oval, or elongated.

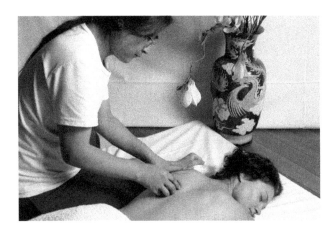

FIG. 26. Massage with stones

To work on muscles, use rounded and oval stones; elongated ones replace finger pressure on the critical points. Stones that are coarser are used for relaxation, to eliminate muscle contracture, and to distribute oil and ensure its absorption.

Using hot stones on points helps to eliminate painful muscle contractions and promotes the elongation of the tendons. When the heat penetrates deeply, it dissolves internal pains of different natures. Moreover, it can be used to treat specific problems such as insomnia, digestive disorders, depression, headaches, bloating, etc.

Among the hard mineral stones, agate can be used and is indicated for bile and liver problems, infection, and acute pain. It calms bile/*tripa* excess due to its cooling characteristic. Turquoise can be used for liver and blood diseases, poisoning, and fever. Pearl is ideal for soothing the nervous system. Jade cures allergies. Pink quartz is useful in cases of skin diseases and joint problems. And hematite is ideal as a cure for lymphatic diseases and joint pain.

Precious and semiprecious stones can be used for massage, although this is not commonly done.

TABLE 8.4
Properties of gemstones

STONE	PROPERTY
Agate	Optimal for problems with bile and inflammation
Amber	Useful for diarrhea, blurred vision, and epilepsy
Citrine quartz	Protects from provocation by external energy and heals injuries
Coral	Used for liver, blood, and nerve disorders
Crystal	Helps fever, inflammation, and mental confusion
Emerald	Protects against negative influences when external therapies are practiced on patients
Hematite	Indicated for lymphatic problems and pain in the bones
Jade	Cures allergies
Lapis lazuli	Protects from animal poisons, snake poisons, and external provocations
Morganite	Optimal in all cases of intoxication or drug abuse
Pearl	Great for nervous system disorders and vision
Rose quartz	Indicated for skin diseases and joint problems
Ruby	Indicated for neurological problems or loss of voice
Turquoise	Indicated for liver and blood problems, poisoning, and fevers

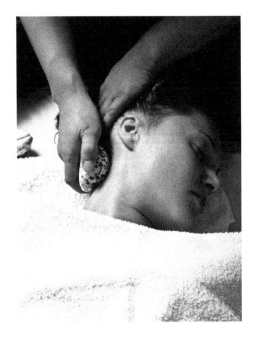

FIG. 27. Massage with shells

Massage with Shells

Massage with shells is a unique technique for the face, performed with the shells of mother-of-pearl. It has a pacifying action on wind/*loong* and on the mind. It stretches and relaxes all the muscles of the face, thus producing an antiwrinkle effect. Mother-of-pearl is considered the most suitable substance for treating neuralgia. The shell of *Ciprea tigris* is used to treat the meridians and disorders of the back muscles.

Stick Massage

Yukchö, or stick massage, is not mentioned in the *Four Tantras* of Traditional Tibetan Medicine (TTM). But it can be considered as part of the external therapies, the last of the four healing methods as illustrated in the third Tree of Sowa Rigpa, the tree of therapy, including diet, behavior, medicine, and external therapies. (See appendix 2 for a detailed history of stick massage.)

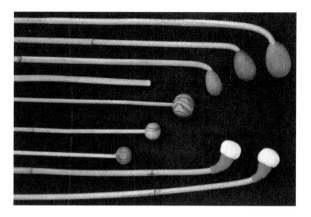

FIG. 28. Yukcho set

The essential tool in this therapy is obviously the stick. Ratnalingpa's manual says that the stick should be bamboo or *Spiraea canescens*, another kind of wood that is very flexible, like willow.[1] The flexibility of the wood is of paramount importance because it prevents possible damage due to tapping on specific points of the body and changes the physiological circulation of wind/*loong* and blood. It also helps to eliminate the waste of the disease easily and rebalance the energy in a very natural way.

The length of the stick should be a cubit, an ancient unit of length based on the length of the forearm of the practitioner from the elbow to the tip of the middle finger, and four fingers. This length enables the therapist to strike with the right degree of strength and also facilitates the percussion. A shorter stick does not produce the necessary strength and a longer one does not strike precisely on the exact point.

It is said that those who practice this form of therapy should have recited the mantra of the tantric deity Hayagriva at least seven hundred thousand times. Hayagriva is the wrathful manifestation, with healing powers, of the buddha of compassion, Avalokitesvara, and is traditionally depicted with a green horse head. Once the recitations of the mantra are completed, we blow on the stick to transmit the power of the mantra. It is particularly important to follow these guidelines, especially when treating

---

[1] It is also possible to use other types of flexible wood.

patients with mental illnesses or diseases that are caused by external provocations.[2] The efficacy of treatment is markedly increased by the power of
the recitations of the mantra.

The tip of the stick should be made in such a way to allow letters of the
mantra to be written on it and a small pouch containing mustard seeds
to be attached. With this pouch at the tip of the stick, contact is made
on the points of the patient's body without damaging the skin or bones
and causing only minimal pain. The other type of stick has an egg-shaped
piece of wood attached at the end instead of the pouch.

The stick is made of *Aquilaria* wood to treat wind/*loong* problems and
of sandalwood for bile/*tripa* problems. This type of stick is heavier; due
to its weight and the depth of its effect, it is more effective on the muscles
or when the problem is serious.

INDICATIONS AND CONTRAINDICATIONS
FOR STICK MASSAGE

Treatment with a stick produces an effect more profound and more powerful than finger pressure. Thanks to the vibrations produced by the stick,
the disorders present in the area in question converge on the treated point
and come out. The concept is similar to that of bloodletting, where after
having assisted the accumulation of impure blood at one point, the practitioner lets the impure blood out of the body.

The points used for stick massage are the same as for other types of
massage.

Stick massage is indicated in the following cases:

Problems related to the head, such as headache and wind/*loong*
    disorder manifested in the head
Deafness and problems in the ears
Stiff or curved neck
Problems with speech articulation
Stiffness or paralysis of limbs
Sadness
Acute back pains

---

[2] External provocations (*don*) from beings without physical bodies that inhabit the environment.

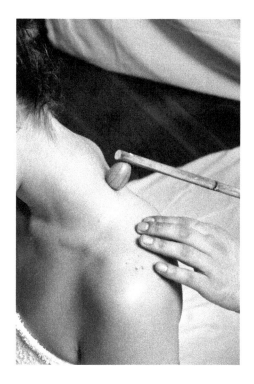

FIG. 29. Stick massage

Feeling of chest tightness

Schizophrenia and madness due to wind/*loong* disorder

Flatulence

Problems in the diaphragm

Liver tumors

Loss of digestive heat

Diseases of the stomach

Excess of gastric mucous

Cramps in the stomach

Intestinal problems due to cold and wind/*loong*

Wind/*loong* disorders in the kidneys

Gynecological diseases and tumor formation or cystitis

Breathing difficulty caused by sorrow and mental problems

Hoarseness

Stammer

These are just some of the problems that can be alleviated by stick massage. It can be helpful for all diseases, provocations, obstacles, and nerve problems that meditation and spiritual practices can sometimes cause.

Points and areas of the body where stick massage is contraindicated:

The central point of the mandala of the elements on the crown of
   the head; can be treated very softly by experienced practitioners,
   but novices should never practice on it
Sense organs
Heart
Breasts and nipples
Points of the face around the mouth
Liver
Spleen
Kidneys
Navel
Genital organs
Clavicle
Kneecap
Popliteal (back of the knee)
Elbows
Lymph nodes
Achilles tendon
Tendons, ligaments, and insertions of muscles and nerves

This therapy is also contraindicated for people with blood disorders, infections, and various kinds of fevers, as well as for infants and during pregnancy.

These instructions should be kept well in the mind to avoid damaging the body and aggravating the disease. It is also necessary not to tap the areas where the protective *la* energy circulates on that day in order to avoid losing this precious energy or changing its location suddenly.

Moxibustion

Moxibustion, or moxa (*metsa* in Tibetan) is an external therapy that uses the application of heat produced by mugwort (*Artemisia vulgaris*) cones or rolled sticks and less common materials like heated stones or wooden sticks on specific and limited areas of the body in order to remove energy blockages, restore proper blood circulation, and relieve pain. The treatment warms and pacifies wind/*loong* and phlegm/*beken*; however, it must be applied cautiously for those of bile/*tripa* humor. Regardless of the typology of the patient, the bile points must be avoided. After treatment they should not drink cold drinks or take cold baths to prevent the heat from dispersing, which would interrupt the energy route stimulated by the moxibustion.

This therapy is indicated in cases of difficult digestion, changes in fire-accompanying wind, swelling caused by phlegm/*beken*, dropsy, headache, excess fluids, osteoarthritis, arthritis, bursitis, and rheumatism. Moreover, moxa is very effective in the treatment of all cold-natured diseases, caused by wind/*loong* and phlegm/*beken*; all neurological problems; channel problems; all lymphatic problems; and problems related to an excess of fluids.

Moxa is easy to apply and very effective when used with discretion. For practitioners of *kunye*, it is very helpful to know the uses of moxa.

The therapeutic action results from the heat produced by burning artemisia and warming the pain points, which promotes the smooth circulation of blood and energy and eliminates energy blocks.

Moxa is applied on wind/*loong* and phlegm/*beken* points, the same as used for massage.

The necessary ingredient is mugwort, which will be collected during the three autumn months, then sun-dried or lightly toasted in a pan. To refine, spread it on a wooden board, mash it with a wooden pestle, and then pour out the dust. What remains will be stored in a wooden box or a bag of leather. Moxa is prepared by rolling and crushing the required amount of mugwort between the palms, trying to give it a rounded shape. Once compressed, press with the fingers to form a cone with a wide base and fine tip for ease of burning. Depending on the problems to be treated, other ingredients can be added to the mugwort. For example, in the case of heart problems we can add some nutmeg.

The cones of mugwort may be of different sizes, depending on the area of the body where they are to be applied. The base of the cones prepared for use on the spine should have the thickness of a thumb joint. For the head, limbs, heart, stomach, small and large intestines, and other organs, the base of the cones should be as small as the tip of the little finger.

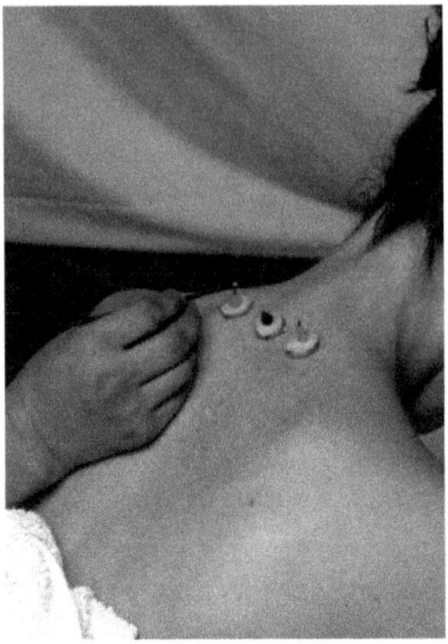

FIG. 30. Cone moxa on ginger slice

In cases of bleeding, the balls should be the size of a marble. To treat the children, the cones must be the size of a pea.

It is important to remember that, to avoid burns and scars, the mugwort cone should be placed on a base for skin protection. We can use a slice of garlic to treat imbalances of wind/*loong* and a slice of ginger for the problems of phlegm/*beken*. And, as explained in further detail below, moxa cones are not placed on the body, but instead are waved above the skin.

Moxa Indications and Contraindications

We may use moxa on *kunye* points, except bile/*tripa* points. We can also apply it to painful points but not inflamed points or areas. That means never to apply moxa where the signs of inflammation (heat, red, swelling and pain) are present.

When a point is cold, swelling, and numb, there is phlegm/*beken* accumulated, while an itchy point means excess of wind/*loong*. In both cases, extended treatment is needed.

To treat a sore area, trace with moxa stick in circles or rays, starting on the most painful point

To treat a sore area, trace with moxa stick in circles or rays, starting on the most painful point, and gradually moving outward.

Moxa is contraindicated in cases of excess heat, bile and liver problems like hepatitis, inflammations, blood diseases (in Sowa Rigpa, blood contains water and fire elements, so treating a blood disease by using moxa may lead to an excess of bile/*tripa*), fever caused by bile/*tripa* and fever in general, and flu.

Furthermore, never use moxa on sense organs (nose, ears, eyes, tongue, lips), the reproductive organs channel, the external genitals (male and female), arteries and veins, or lymphatic glands.

Four Levels of Moxa Application

According to Sowa Rigpa, moxa with mugwort can be applied in four different levels of decreasing intensity; cooking, burning, heating, and alarming.

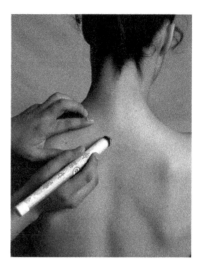

FIG. 31. Waving a moxa stick over points on the back.

"Cooking" level—Application of moxa on the same point for twenty-one times in a row. Let the cone burn to the end, then light another, until twenty-one cones are burned out. Skin and flesh at that point become as if they were "cooked." This level is indicated in cases of abscesses, tumors, or serious conditions of cold and phlegm/*beken*. To prevent burning, use a wood support.

"Burning" level—Apply moxa cones fifteen consecutive times. This is indicated for depressive disorders, problems of excessive wind/*loong* in the heart, and lymphatic and phlegm/*beken* problems. It is also advisable, in this case, to use a wooden support.

"Heating" level—Application of moxa cones seven times. This level is indicated to treat wind/*loong* imbalances, diseases caused by bacteria, constipation, and urinary disorders.

"Alarming" level—Technique used in children. Moxa or an incense stick is applied to the point to be treated gradually, until the child reacts to the heat.

All these methods derived from Tibet and were used by Tibetan doctors centuries ago.

An optimal method, applied today, is using mugwort sticks to heat the skin without touching or burning. Light a moxa stick and hover it over the point so that the receiver does not receive too-intense heat. Then remove the stick and bring it back over the point for the necessary number of times.

The moxa stick can be used in three different ways: fixed over the point, circling over the point clockwise and counterclockwise, and moving in and out over the point.

Types of Moxa

There are several types of moxa, depending on the materials used, for example: mugwort (*Artemisia*), wooden, Mongolian, golden needle, metal, etc.

The particular types of moxa sessions are described in more detail below.

MOXA WITH MUGWORT CONES AND STICKS: *DRA ME*

It is necessary to identify the point to be treated precisely. Apply a drop of garlic juice or other sticky substance on the point so that the *Artemisia* cone adheres to the skin. Light the cone with incense, blowing gently. Let the cone burn down and remove it at the end.

The mugwort cone can also be placed on a slice of garlic over the point, which is very useful for problems of wind/*loong*. It is best when the cone burns down with a crackling sound. Then remove the ashes and the garlic slice. Finish the treatment by applying a small amount of salted butter on the point.

As a base for the mugwort cone, you can also use a thin piece of wood or a piece of cardboard with a small hole in the middle to let the heat pass through. On points with hair, use a round wooden base with a handle, such as a wooden spoon with a single hole.

For a softer moxa and to prevent scarring, use the rolled moxa stick, moving it toward and away from the point to be treated repeatedly.

After the treatment, patient should walk around and avoid drinking cold drinks for the rest of the day. No cold showers for two days after the moxa.

MOXA WITH GOLDEN NEEDLE: *SER ME*

Practice solely on the central point of the crown after having located the point precisely. Put a ball of good-quality mugwort on the upper end of the golden acupuncture needle (silver can also be used). Adhere closely a piece of wood or very thin cardboard with a small hole in the center over the crown point as a protective base and insert the needle tip in point number one of the crown by a few millimeters, just deep enough for the needle to remain standing on its own. Light the mugwort and let it burn down. If the mugwort has difficulty burning, blow on it gently from time to time. The needle should be withdrawn from the point only when it has cooled.

Moxa with golden needles is effective for curing psychiatric diseases, such as schizophrenia and madness.

WOODEN MOXA: *SHING ME*

The mugwort cone should be placed in the center of a wooden slat. Light the cone and let it burn down completely. Repeat three or five times.

Another way to do this is to grind the cone to a powder and mix in small equal parts of calcite, *Indian robbia* and *Piper longum*. Place a thin layer of powder over the point to be treated and cover with a red cloth and a thin piece of untreated wood.

This is a particularly effective method to treat serum problems, the presence of synovial liquid in the joints, arthritis, and gout. The calcite absorbs the heat and sends it deeper into the point.

WATER MOXA: *CHU ME*

Sprinkle calcite or lime powder on the chosen point. Wet the powder with a drop of water. Place the mugwort cone on top of the dampened powder, light it, and let it burn down.

As an alternative, a moxa stick can be used. In Sowa Rigpa, water moxa is suitable for digestive problems and meteorism.

MOXA WITH METAL INSTRUMENT: *TEL ME*

Place a metal instrument made of gold, silver, copper, or iron into hot embers until it is glowing.

It is necessary to protect the skin on and around the point to be treated and to avoid deep burns. This can be done by placing a piece of fabric with a hole in the middle over the point. Heat the point with the hot tip of the metal instrument. To avoid burning the skin, put a thin piece of wood under the fabric or just use the wood as a base with a hole, letting the heat pass through but avoid touching the skin directly with the hot metal tool.

HORN MOXA: *RA TSUG*

Moxibustion can be done with the point of an animal's horn that has been rounded off with a stone. Bring the heated horn close to the points that are manifesting lymphatic problems, edema, or accumulation of liquids. To avoid unnecessary burns, use a protective base and know that is enough to heat the point without burning it.

STONE MOXA: *DO TSUG*

Heat in an oven or on the fire some slightly elongated river pebbles or small stones and place them on the points. A stone with a hole in the center can be used as a frame to avoid burning the skin. This type of moxa can also be practiced using a heated calcite cone, placing it close to the point and then removing it many times. Place the cone directly on the point only when it is not too hot.

MOXA WITH A SMALL WOODEN BRANCH: *SHING TSUG*

Rub a sandalwood branch together with another sandalwood stick, creating heat with the friction, or simply warm up the wood over a small flame. Put it warm on specific points.

Mongolian Moxa: Horme

Horme or *hor gyi me tsa* is one of the many techniques of moxibustion that originated in Mongolia very early. It was integrated as an external therapy in Tibetan medicine, with some doctors claiming to have invented it. Most probably, *horme* first appeared in Mongolia, while the theory and practice have been developed over the ages by traditional Tibetan medicine.

The name is derived from the Horo Tibetan kingdom (*Hos ro*), one of the twelve minor kingdoms into which the territory of Tibet was divided in 2000 B.C.E.

The first traces of this external therapy are found in the most ancient treatise on Tibetan medicine, *Bum Shi, The Four Thousand Ways of Medicine*, transcriptions of medical teachings by the Bon master Sherab Miwoche (1999–1917 B.C.E.) written by his son Che bu Tri shi (Tib. *DPyat Bu Khri shes*), the first Tibetan doctor.

In *The Root Tantra*, the first of the *Four Tantras, Gyud Shi*, of Tibetan medical science, *horme* is illustrated in the tree of therapy as the best external therapy for imbalances of wind/*loong*, along with *kunye* massage.

THERAPEUTIC EFFECTS OF *HORME*

Horme decreases wind/*loong* excess in order to restore energetic balance. Heat applied to the points warms the cold nature of wind/*loong*, and the heavy potentiality of oil compensates for its light nature, thus rebalancing it.

Horme is the most effective Tibetan external therapy for the treatment of mental and emotional derangement, to calm and to relax tension and stress. In traditional Tibetan medicine, *horme* is also indicated for treating pathologies such as *nying loong*, disorder of *loong* in the heart; *pho loong*, disorder of wind/*loong* in the stomach; *chin loong*, disorder of *loong* in the liver, and all disorders of the five types of wind/*loong*.

THE PRACTICE OF *HORME*

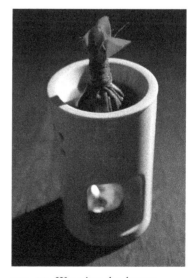

The ancient technique is to immerse little pieces of felt that have been exposed to the heat of the sun or fire for a very long time, in warm sesame oil. Once the felt is well-warmed and oil-soaked, fit the pieces over the kidneys and the joints of the hands and limbs to cure cold problems. More recently, small compresses preferably made of red cotton, representing the fire element, and filled with specific herbs or seeds are used. These can be immersed in warm sesame oil and applied on the wind/*loong* points to pacify its excess.

FIG. 32. Warming the *horme* pouch

HORME PRESCRIPTIONS

The mixture of the herbs contained in the small compresses may vary depending on the desired effects.

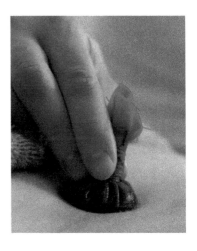

The classic formula to pacify a strong wind/*loong* excess, as may occur after a patient delivers a baby or in the case of shock or family tragedy, after strong bleeding, fainting episodes, or in the case of postsurgical convalescence, is as follows:

Small *horme* compresses are applied on all the wind/*loong* points. These should contain fresh aniseed, nutmeg, slices of fresh ginger, and fresh garlic in

FIG. 33. *Horme* application

equal proportions and well blended with the help of a mortar and pestle.

Doctor Ju Mipham, one of the greatest Tibetan scholars of philosophy, astrology, and medicine of the nineteenth century, author of fourteen texts on these sciences, was famous for his personal style in the preparation of remedies that always had to contain five substances: nutmeg, garlic, ginger, aniseed, and sandalwood. In his text *Collected Works on Tibetan Medicine*, he indicates the following prescriptions for *horme*:

> *Loong* disorder: compress with equal parts of aniseed and nutmeg in warm sesame oil
> *Loong/tripa* disorder: compress with equal parts of aniseed, garlic, and sandalwood powder in warm olive oil or ghee
> *Loong/beken* disorder: compress with equal parts of aniseed and ginger in warm sesame oil

More specific prescriptions, found in the other sources, are as follows:

> *Horme* for the ears to calm the body and the mind: soak two little wads of felt in warm sesame oil and insert them in the auricular tubes
> *Horme* for blood circulation problems: after a *kunye* massage of the affected areas performed with sesame oil mixed with turmeric powder, prepare *horme* compresses with sesame seeds, turmer-

CASE STUDY 3

An Italian man suffered from sharp chest pain accompanied by a sensation as if he couldn't breathe. It was similar to a panic attack, and he got very emotional and nervous and couldn't sleep. His biomedical physicians examined his heart and checked for acidity and other conditions using various other diagnostic tests, with no clear results. I diagnosed him with a *nying loong*, a wind/*loong* disturbance in the heart, and recommended the external therapy of *horme* on the point (*kar nag sang*) in the center of the chest as well as the heart mandala points, the points in four directions around the left nipple. After receiving and learning the technique, the patient continued to practice on himself at home. After seven days, the condition was resolved.

ic, and ginger in equal parts. Apply them on the center of the sole when circulatory problems affect the leg, or place them in the center of the palm when the problem affects the arm; or on whichever point where a circulatory stagnation may be present.

Horme after delivery of a baby: to help the new mother to recover her energies and to avoid wind/*loong* disorder, compresses with cloves, sesame seeds, garlic, and ginger in equal parts should be applied on the points of descending wind/*loong*; on the internal and external gates of the head; on the first, sixth, and seventh Tibetan vertebrae[3]; and on the center of the pubic bone, where pain is perceived when pressure is exerted. The application of *horme* on descending wind/*loong* points may also accelerate delivery when problems occur.

Horme with stones: in case of bone or muscular pains, muscle or tendon stiffness, and cold retention, boil a piece of felt, which has been aged in the sun, in sesame oil. Once the felt has cooled down but is still warm, it can be applied on the affected point. Heat a river stone in an oven or near the fire and place the heated stone over the felt. This procedure can be applied on the wind/*loong* points, on the joints, and on the vertebrae.

---

[3] In Sowa Rigpa, the seventh cervical vertebra is considered the first Tibetan vertebrae point. Palpated downward from this, there 24 Tibetan vertebrae points along the vertebral spinous processes.

Unfavorable Days for Moxa Treatments

Never apply moxa, bloodletting, or surgical procedures in the area where the protective *la* energy is located on the day of treatment according to the lunar calendar; and on the 1st, 6th, 15th, 18th, 20th, and 30th lunar calendar day.

Soft moxa or other soft therapies like massage and baths can be used any day, but invasive and strong therapies like bloodletting, acupuncture, and surgery should be avoided on unfavorable days.

Compress Therapy

Compresses, filled with medicinal ingredients, salt, or stones, may be applied on specific body points. This therapy enhances the effects of *kunye*. The compresses give instant relief when applied to painful points.

Depending on the nature of the problems, different materials and herbs are used. Compresses may be applied hot or cold.

Cold Compresses

These need to be filled with materials having a cold nature, like metals, agate, or river stones, and are suitable for:

Fever caused by trauma or accident
Sharp pain caused by fever and worsened by inappropriate diet and lifestyle (put a cold water bottle under the armpits or between the thighs, or simply apply some cold water)
Strong and chronic fever (put cold water on the areas affected)
Sharp intestinal pain (apply a cold water bottle on the area, adding white aconitum and symplocos to the water)
Sharp pain caused by fever (put cold river stones on the affected area)
Excess heat in the liver and excess bile/*tripa* (apply flat agate slices on the liver points)
Nosebleed (apply cold water on the forehead and on the occipital bone)

CASE STUDY 4

An East Asian man, age 36, suffered from severe recurring abdominal pain and sweating. He went three times to the hospital for various types of diagnostic tests, but they were inconclusive.

His pulse and urine all indicated heat pathology, *tsawa* (Tib. *tsha ba*). I recommended him to use a cold stone compress on the abdomen. After a few days the pain completely disappeared and didn't return.

Hangover (apply a cold water bottle on the temporal points and both sides of the neck)

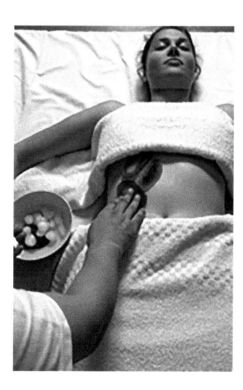

FIG. 34. Cold agate compress on liver points.

Hot Compresses

Warm compresses are suitable for all the following cases:

- Muscular pain caused by cold weather (cut fresh ginger in little pieces, wrap in a cotton cloth, warm with steam, apply to the affected area)
- Asthma and respiratory problems (make two compresses filled with broken petals of white gentiana; warm them and place one on the chest and the other on the back, covering the area of the lungs)
- Difficult digestion caused by a combined imbalance of wind/*loong* and phlegm/*beken* (warm hands and place them on the stomach's critical points)
- Blood circulation problems caused by wounds (place a warm stone on the affected area)
- Sharp kidney pain caused by cold weather and urinary blockage (apply dried barley left over from brewing Tibetan beer [*chang*] to the affected area)
- Postdelivery intestine and lumbar pain (place a natural cloth bag filled with heated sand and a little alcohol on the painful area)
- Intestinal colic caused by stomach inflammations (soak in water *althea rosea*, rhubarb, and *symplocos* leaves; warm up and apply)
- Cold-natured diseases (heat a brick or other clay object and place it on the affected area)
- Sharp pain caused by wind/*loong* disorders (soak a piece of woolen felt with warm oil or warm up a river stone, wet it with warm oil, and put it on the area)
- Cold in the stomach, small intestine, and colon (warm hands and place them on the area)
- Cold in the kidneys and on the hips (place on the area a piece of animal fur [traditionally a wolf's fur, but the fur of any animal will do])
- Joint swelling due to an excess of liquids (heat some small river stones, spread a little alcohol on them, and apply to joints)
- Acute pain caused by fever related to wind/*loong* disorder (apply white quartz or warm stone, wetted with a little red wine)
- Excess of liquid and lymphatic problems of the limbs (heat up sheep dung with a little red wine and apply to the swollen part)

Do not use compresses for anemia, infectious diseases and infections in general, leprosy, poisoning, intoxication, edema with fever, or pimples. And in any case, do not apply compresses immediately after eating.

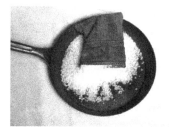

FIG. 35. Hot salt compress

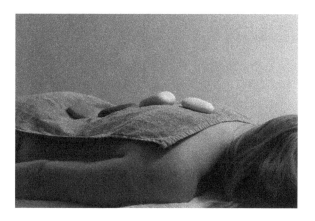

FIG. 36. Hot stone compress

CASE STUDY 5

A 23-year-old Italian woman had recurring uterine cysts and painful menstruation. She had the cysts surgically removed, but they grew back. The only other possible solutions suggested by her gynecologists were additional surgeries or possibly pregnancy.

Her Tibetan medical diagnosis was *tren (skran)* disorder, benign growths that originate from indigestion and the blood metabolic process. As a therapy, I recommended that she take two pills of the herbal formula Kyuru 25, three times per day, and apply a hot compress two to three days per week. After three months, she had an additional scan and the growths were completely gone.

Cupping Therapy

Cupping, in Tibetan *me bum*, literally means "vase of fire." Traditionally, a little copper or glass bowl is used. Copper is believed to have absorbing properties, thus helping negative energies to come out of the body, but silver and brass share the same properties. Nowadays, glass cups are widely used.

We may use this therapy, also known as "the therapy with Buddha's nectar vase," to get rid of an excess of wind/*loong*, bile/*tripa*, or phlegm/*beken* accumulated in a specific area. Thus, cupping promotes a harmonic flow of energies. It is suitable in all the following cases:

Acute pains on the upper part of the back, caused by blood or
    wind/*loong* dysfunctions
Combinations of blood and wind/*loong* diseases, manifested in the
    upper part of the body
Blockages in the upper part of the body
Wind/*loong* disorders
Hip sprain
Oppressive chest pain
Respiratory disorders and hyperventilation

Cupping can be applied to treat points below the cltavicle and to all the painful points or areas suffering from wind/*loong* or blood disorders.

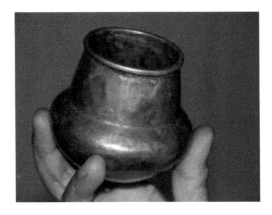

FIG. 37. Traditional Tibetan copper cup

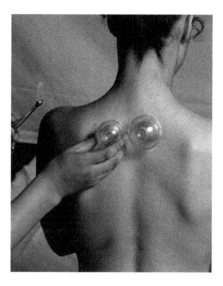

FIG. 38. Cupping alternative

Suction is created using heat (fire) and the cup is placed on the point for fifteen to twenty minutes.

Once the cup has been removed, the skin may show different reactions according to the humors. Open pores and straight hair mean that a wind/*loong* problem has been solved. Pale and swollen skin means that the problem is related to phlegm/*beken*. A dark red mark indicates that bile/*tripa* is the cause of the problem.

Use larger cups to treat a bigger area and smaller cups for the joints.

A cupping session followed by bloodletting is called "wet cupping," and it is good for treating acute pain caused by blood disorders. Cupping used alone is called "dry cupping" and is good for acute pains and pain caused by wind/*loong* disorders.

Cupping Indications

Stiffness and tensed muscles of the neck, back, and trapezius
Cough: place the cups on both sides of the neck and on both sides of the upper part of the sternum

Asthma attacks: place two cups, one on the chest, on the lung area, and the other on the back, at the same height and always in correspondence with the first one. Following oil application, move the two cups over the anterior and posterior bronchi-pulmonary areas

Diaphragm spasms and hiccups: place two cups, one on the sternum at nipple level and the other on the spine, at the same height

Intercostals pain: move the cup over the ribs

Meteorism, menstrual pain, and diarrhea: apply one cup below the navel

Sciatica: place and move the cup on gluteus mandala points

Snake bite: sck out the poison by applying the cup over the bite, to prevent poison diffusion in the body

Cupping Contraindications

Pregnancy
Infectious diseases
Pain and swelling caused by inflammatory conditions
Underweight
Bleeding wounds
Sense organs

Horn Therapy

Horn therapy is similar to using cups, except it uses an animal's horn instead. In Tibetan, *ngab ra*, the sucking horn, is used to make the wind/*loong* leave the body from specific points. The horn has to be short, for instance, from a cow or ox, and a hole should be made in the tip.

Place the horn standing on its base where the treatment is needed. Connect a rubber hose with a syringe to the horn's tip. With the syringe, suck out the air from the horn and immediately tie the cable to stop air from entering and create a vacuum to help the wind/*loong* come out of the body. During this time, apply wind/*loong* oil on the crown and soles.

This treatment is suitable for poisonous snake bites, wind/*loong* disorders, tumors, gout, arthritis, excess of fluids and serum problems,

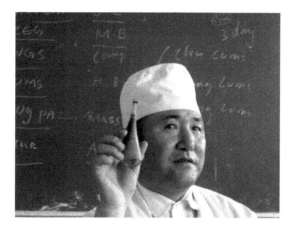

FIG. 39. Dr. Padma from Xining Tibetan Medicine Hospital
showing the horn used in horn therapy

and illnesses of bacteriological origin. Contraindications are the same
as for cupping.

Fumigation Therapy

This therapy, in Tibetan called *loong dug*, is based on the sense of smell
and uses the smoke of particular medicinal substances burning on amber.
Allow the smoke to reach the receiver's body entirely. Alternatively, the
receiver may inhale the smoke.

The smoke from roasted barley powder relieves wind/*loong* imbalances.
We may use the powder by itself or combined with agarwood (*Aquilaria
agallocha*). It is recommended to burn these substances or good-quality
agarwood incense in the treatment room.

Fumigation therapy is suitable for dizziness, fainting, nausea, headache, weakness, severe hemorrhages, postpartum recovery, and postsurgical recovery.

Smoke therapy with rhododendron or peach flowers can be done at
home, or the flowers can be steamed and used as a compress on the body
to help prevent flu and other contagious illnesses.

Bath Therapy

Bath therapy in Tibetan is called *chu lum*. This therapy is specifically connected to the water element and uses thermal spring water that naturally
contains therapeutic properties or water in which medicinal herbs have
been boiled. Water or steam can be used.

Bath therapy is usually very effective in treating neurological and wind/
loong disorders. Water relaxes tense and stiff nerves, tendons, and ligaments.

Bath Therapy Indications

The various kinds of bath and steam therapies are fundamentally similar,
and all are suitable for the following cases:

Muscle, tendon, ligament, and limb stiffness
Limb paralysis
Abscesses
Contagious muscle tissue infection
Chronic stomach ulcers
Recent wound
Swelling and ulcerations containing liquids
Menstrual problems caused by wind/*loong* and phlegm/*beken*
    disorders
Curvature of the spine, such as kyphosis
Swollen muscles and bones due to an excess of liquids
Any kind of wind/*loong* disorder

Bath Therapy Contraindications

Fever caused by infectious illness
Fever worsened by inappropriate diet and lifestyle
High fever
Swelling caused by phlegm/*beken*
Physical weakness
Lack of appetite

Types of Bath Therapy

THERMAL WATERS BATH

Thermal spring water is a natural phenomenon on our planet. This water has a particularly powerful therapeutic effect and is easily accessible for everybody.

Calcite and slaked lime
Calcite and sulphur
Calcite and mineral exudates (mineral of pitch)
Calcite, sulphur, and rocks sweating
Calcite, sulphur, mineral exudates, and realgar

Before the bath, protect with a white or any natural cloth the testicles, navel, knees, elbows, and cardiac area. People with gout should cover the affected limbs. When the water is pure, the patient should drink two or three glasses before soaking. Moreover, according to Sowa Rigpa, it is advisable to wet the chest, elbows, and knees before entering the water.

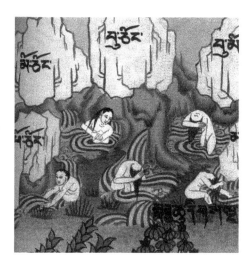

FIG. 40. Bathing in mineral springs

Enter to the water gradually, first with the feet; wait a while, then enter up to the knees and wait again; then finally and gradually immerse the body completely.

After the bath the patient should wear a thick bathrobe, in order to facilitate sweating.

The bath sessions should progressively last longer, and the duration should be set according to the person's constitution. A person with a strong constitution is allowed to bathe every day and for up to three weeks, even if affected by a severe illness. A person of medium constitution or a wind typology should bathe every second day.

A medical examination is necessary before starting the therapy, so that problems will not be aggravated. Gradual treatment is very important. Progressively increase the duration of the bath and, once the maximum has been reached, gradually reduce the duration until the end of the cycle.

FIVE NECTARS MEDICINAL BATH

Sowa Rigpa medicinal baths are usually prepared with five herbs called "the five nectars," *dul tsi nga lum*:

Rhododendron flowers—softens the skin
Salt cedar—eliminates toxic substances from bones; the entire plant
     is used
Ephedra—Reinvigorates the body; use the stem only
White artemisia—balances the elements' energies; the entire plant
     is used
Juniper—known as the "plant with one hundred healing properties"
     and as a general tissue tonic; leaves and small branches are used

These five plants strengthen the body and balance the energies; thus, the five nectars bath is recommended for both unhealthy and healthy people.

To increase the efficacy and strengthen the effects we can add other ingredients, such as the "five roots":

Peucedanum officinale
Common Solomon's seal, *Polygonatum X hybridum*

Asparagus racemosus
Mirabilis jalapa
Tribulus terrestris

For serum-related problems, sap of *Shorea robusta, Cassia angustifolia* (senna), and *Abelmoschus esculentus* may be added. Never add to the decoction toxic, purgative, or emetic substances.

Pour the heated decoction into the bath water. As an alternative, simply wrap the ingredients in a cloth and put the pouch into the bath water.

The procedure for bathing in the five nectars is the same as for bathing in thermal waters: cover the sensitive areas with white cloth, enter the water gradually and slowly, wait a few minutes before the next stage. Entering gradually avoids sudden changes in blood circulation, in heartbeat, and in the way the wind/*loong* energy flows. Entering the water too quickly leads to hyperventilation, dizziness, and nausea. Elderly or overweight people should bathe only below the heart area, in order to protect their heart. A person in a good physical condition is allowed to take two baths a day. A weak person or one suffering from a chronic disease should bathe only once a day, although the treatment cycle should last longer than usual, up to four weeks.

The right amount and frequency of bathing depend on the patient's physical strength and the seriousness of the disease. One bath a day may be enough. After the bath a *kunye* massage is recommended.

The bath temperature should increase gradually day by day and once the maximum temperature is reached, it should then gradually decrease until the end of the therapy. Risks rise with the temperature and only gradual increases can reduce them. Dipping straight into the water at 104–107°F/40–42°C could be very risky, especially when bile/*tripa* problems are present.

Precautions

During the bath therapy cycle, the patient should avoid cold drinks, washing in cold water, lying down or sleeping on humid ground or in humid locations, wearing lightweight clothing, not wearing enough clothing, eating food difficult to digest, and walking barefoot or without clothes.

Treatment of the Energy Channels

In the Tibetan medicine view of the body, there are thirteen internal energy channels or meridians that are connected to the internal organs and six external channels or meridians with lines located along the limbs.

External Channels

There are three pairs of superficial channels:

Two channels called *buguchen*, tubular channels. *Buguchen* means big tube. These are involved in the pathologies of the sciatic nerve, senses organs, memory, and arms.

Two channels called *jache* channels of paralysis. The treatment of these meridians is particularly indicated in cases of paralysis, whatever the cause.

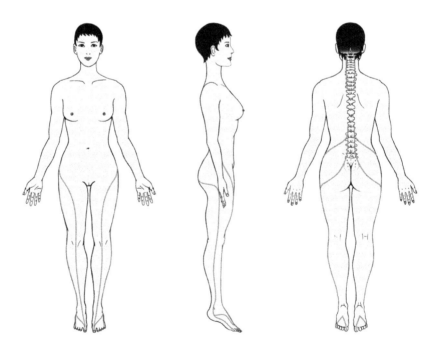

FIG. 41. Buguchen channels

Two channels called *ratna*, precious channels. Through these channels flows the energy related to wind/*loong*, called by Tibetans
"the precious energy."

THE *BUGUCHEN* CHANNELS

The *buguchen* channel comes out from the brain and branches into two
channels that go down either side of the spine, then continue along the
outside of each leg. Each channel branches again at the ankle, with one
branch going through the big toe and the other going through the little
toe; then the two branches meet again in the middle of the sole.

The other channel comes out at the fourteenth vertebra, one on the
left side and the other on the right side. It crosses the gluteus diagonally
and goes through the front of the leg (thigh) and knee, then runs along
the inner side of the kneecap and along the tibia (shin bone). It goes
through the big toe and joins with the other two branches in the middle
of the sole.

THE *JACHE* CHANNELS

The *jache* channels come out either side of the back of the head, go along
the tops of the shoulders and down the arms, and end in the palms.

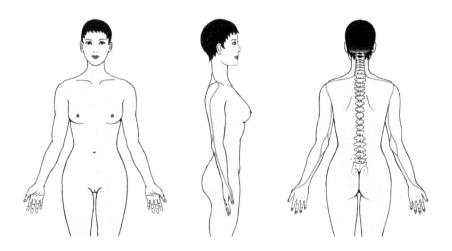

FIG. 42. Jache channels

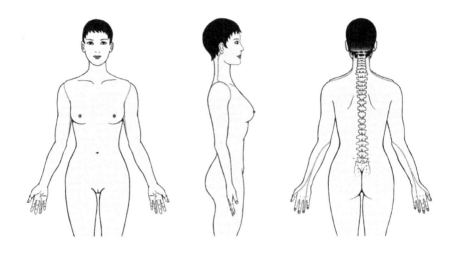

FIG. 43. Ratna channels

THE *RATNA* CHANNELS

These channels run from the lower part of the ears to the cheeks. There
they fork. One branch goes down the lower jaw and regulates mastication.
The other branch goes behind the clavicle, then down the armpit to the
arm; it crosses the deltoid muscles and then runs along the elbow to the
wrist. At the wrist it forks again, and one branch goes through the thumb;
the other branch goes through the ring finger. Both branches rejoin in the
middle of the palm.

Massage of these channels is very useful to balance the energies that
flow through them and to restore the proper function of the organs.

Internal Channels

There are thirteen internal channels originatig from the area of the cer-
ebellum, running through the neck, and then linking up with the internal organs and coming together in the genital/sexual channels. They

are differentiated based on the humor they are associated with and their function.

Four channels of wind are related to the heart and small intestine, and regulate the humor wind/*loong* in these organs.

Four channels of bile are connected to the lung, colon, liver, and gall bladder, and regulate the bile/*tripa* (or metabolic heat, *me drod*) in these organs.

Four channels of phlegm are connected to the stomach, spleen, kidneys, and bladder, and regulate the phlegm/*beken* in these organs.

The thirteenth channel is connected to the ovaries in women and to the seminal vesicles in men, and regulates the three humors in these three organs.

The internal meridians can be treated via so-called target or therapeutic points, connected with the particular channel or organ.

Therapeutic Points in Sowa Rigpa

Points (*sang mig*) are considered in Sowa Rigpa as secret targets. There are two types of points in traditional Tibetan medicine: those affected by a particular problem, i.e., painful points, and specific points.

Painful points are easy to find because they are painful and denote the physical presence of a disorder to be treated, for example with massage. Specific points are very important, although they may not be painful. Each has a specific function and position. The practitioner can cure various diseases using the techniques of rotation, pressure, and heat of the points, as each is directly connected to a specific organ and its respective humor.

The points are also an important diagnostic tool. By checking the appearance of the skin on the point, its temperature, and its sensitivity to pressure, one can discover the underlying pathology.

The specific points are used in Sowa Rigpa for external therapies and are divided into:

Me sang: points for the application of moxa. Moxibustion, commonly called moxa, warms the wind and blood, stimulates and dispels stagnation of blood and wind/*loong*, and eliminates moisture. The heat dissolves and speeds up the circulation of blood and fluids.

TABLE 8.5

Table for verification of the points

HUMOR	APPEARANCE OF THE SKIN	SKIN TEMPERATURE	PERCEPTION OF THE POINT	PAIN OF THE POINT
Wind/*loong*	Blue or gray, with hair standing, it means that the pores are open.	Neither hot nor cold	Soft, empty	Mixed feelings, itching, tingling, and pain together
Bile/*tripa*	Red or brown	Hot	Hard	Acute
Phlegm/ *beken*	Soft, white, puffy	Cold	The point does not return immediately after pressure	Dull

Tar sang: points for bloodletting. Bloodletting draws out impure blood and the negative energies after they are concentrated in one area. The process reduces the heat in the blood.

Yuk sang: points for the use of stick therapy. The stick stimulates the points through vibration. It is faster and more powerful than moxa. The flexibility of the wood is very important in unblocking the channels.

Thur sang: points for acupuncture. Acupuncture concentrates the heat and removes it and the negative energies. Through the needles one can also transmit heat to the points by applying moxa to the needle or transmit cold with a frozen needle. Acupuncture is good for everyone.

Specific tpoints for massage (*sang nye*) are those suitable for moxibustion, with the addition of some items listed for bloodletting and acupuncture.

The effectiveness of a treatment of the points depends on the stage of the physical problem; treatment is more efficient if done when the initial symptoms appear. All the points are connected to the channels through which energy flows, on three levels: organs, humors, and elements. Treating the point treats all the levels, not only the physical part.

The points are treated with the techniques of rotation, pressure, and heating. The degree of pressure to use at each point depends on the sensitivity of the patient. Some points are naturally very sensitive, such as those located in the fontanel of the head.

When the practitioner chooses the points to be treated, he or she has to find the source of the disorder in order to use an appropriate technique. If the pain is in the chest, there is a surplus of wind/*loong* energy to be discharged with massage techniques. For example, for headache, the practitioner will massage the points located on the head. But if the pain is caused by an imbalance of bile, the therapist will have to massage the points of the back connected with this humor and the liver and gall bladder points. If the pain is in the back, the therapist must determine whether it is caused by trauma, osteoarthritis, or osteoporosis. The latter cases must be treated very gently by applying heat.

Sowa Rigpa uses maps of the points located on the head, face, front and back of the body, and limbs. *The points located in the head and back are more sensitive and more important.*

To locate the points, it is necessary to remember that the seventh cervical vertebra is considered the first vertebra point. Palpated downward

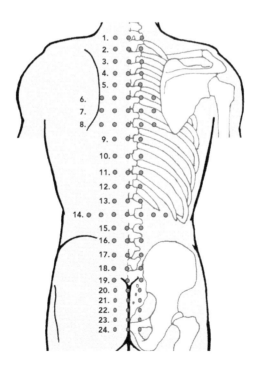

FIG. 44. Points of the back

from this, there are all together twenty-four points along the vertebral spinous processes. For each vertebra, the lateral points are two finger widths to either side of the central point at the spine. Treatment can be performed on these three points found at each vertebral level.

The points on the back and their associated disorders:
1. Point of wind/*loong* (seventh cervical vertebra): mood swings, insomnia, fatigue, and pain in the shoulders.

2. Point of bile/*tripa*: hypertension, bile and gall bladder disorders, high blood pressure, and jaundice in the eyes.

3. Point of phlegm/*beken*: heart and lung disorders, lack of appetite, vomiting, hoarseness caused by alcohol, voice stress; heart-lungs and small circulation problems. Treated to recharge the lungs and to detoxify from smoking.

4. Point of the anterior part of the lungs: breathing problems, pain in the upper back, cough with catarrh caused by phlegm in the lungs.

5. Point of the posterior part of the lungs: lung inflammation related to excess heat (bile/*tripa*), cough with yellowish catarrh (bile/*tripa* in the lungs). In case of pain or tension in the lower back, treat this point gently if unsure of the diagnosis.

6. Point of the aorta: anxiety, emotional problems, insomnia, depression, sadness, fatigue, breathing disorders caused by the heart; bent back caused by mental disorder, madness.

7. Point of the heart: emotional heart problems, madness, lack of memory, fainting and stiff limbs caused by shock and depression as wind/*loong* energy flows through the aorta and heart.

8. Point of the diaphragm: body contractions, pain in the front part of the body, pain in the lower part of the chest, dry vomiting, hiccups, burping, flatulence, hyperkyphosis, difficulty standing straight, dim eyesight. The eyes are related to the liver, which is located close to the diaphragm; this is why this point is important for eye problems. Treating it can cure excess phlegm/*beken*.

9. Point of the kiver: hepatic disorders, problems related to the blood since the liver gathers the blood. Treating this point can cure vomiting (with empty stomach), poisoning caused by food or drugs, eye diseases, myopia, acidity caused by alcohol, cirrhosis, liver cancer, and obesity.

10. Point of the gall bladder: vomit with bile, eye jaundice, calculus (gravel stones) and digestion disorders; bitter taste in the mouth, fever, and gall bladder disorder.

11. Point of the spleen and pancreas: constipation, intestinal rumbling, cracked lips, dry and cracked skin, and spleen disorder. Intestinal rumbling can originate in different organs such as the spleen, liver, small intestine, large intestine, and colon. Treating the point of the spleen helps only if the problem is located on the left side of the abdominal region.

12. Point of the stomach: digestion disorders, problems related to food absorption, stomach cancer, ulcer, gastritis, and lack of metabolic heat needed for digestion.

13. Point of the seminal vesicles, prostate, testicles or ovaries: menstrual disorders, mental and memory disorders, lack of desire, uterine cancer, abnormal sperm production, premature ejaculation, abnormal flow of menstrual blood, too frequent menstruation, anxiety associated with menstruation.

14. Point of the kidneys: problems in the cold parts of the body, kidney dysfunction, sexual problems, lack of desire, impotence, frequent urination, pain in the lumbar area, ear buzzing after alcohol or sexual excesses, and kidney weakness. However, if the patient hears voices, the points to be treated are different, since this is the symptom of unbalanced wind/*loong*. The kidneys are connected with sexual activities.

15. A general point for all internal organs: working a lot with this point helps balance the energies.

16. Point of the colon: colon diseases, intestinal rumbling. If the rumblings are in the upper abdominal region, the internal gas is produced in the spleen and will take time to be discharged. If the rumblings are in the lower part of the abdominal region, the gas is produced in the colon and can be quickly discharged.

17. Point of the small intestine: diarrhea, flatulence, and intestinal tumors.

18. Point of the urinary bladder: calculus stones in bladder and kidneys, frequent urination, cystitis (in this case use decoction rather than oil), and prostate disorders.

19. Point of ovulation and sperm production: menstrual disorders, premature ejaculation, prostate disorders, lack of menstrual flow, and amenorrhea.

20. Descending wind/*loong* (downward wind): constipation and flatulence. This point assists in the discharge of intestinal gases.

21. Descending wind/*loong*: problems related to feces, urine, menstrual blood, sperm, and ejaculation.

22. Descending wind/*loong*: hemorrhoids.

23. Descending wind/*loong*: genital disorders; swollen or contracted testicles.

24. Descending wind/*loong*: difficulty related to orgasms, sexual activity, and ejaculation.

The Protective Energy *La* and Its Cycle

A unique energetic aspect that Tibetan medicine and astrology share is the protective energy or *la*. *La* is the pure energy of the five elements, and it is the vital essence of an individual's consciousness.

Astrology is deeply connected with *la* and certain other aspects of the theory and practice of Tibetan medicine. It originated in Tibet a few thousand years ago, as a native system, not influenced by ideas imported from neighboring countries. And it developed from the observation of the movement of the stars and other heavenly bodies (referred as superior astrology); of clouds, snow, and wind (intermediate astrology); and the behavior of birds, characteristics of trees, forests, lakes, and the formation of ice on lakes and rivers. This ancient body of knowledge has grown over the centuries to become a true and proper astrological system. As the cycles of years, months, days of the waxing and waning phases of the moon, and the movements of the sun were included, it also became possible to express them with greater precision and clarity.

Tibetan scholars observed the reciprocal interaction between the external world and the human body and the influence that the outside world has on any human being based on the fact that the external environment and all living things are made from the same energy, that of the five elements. And this knowledge has become the common heritage of the astrological and medical systems. For example, imbalances of the three humors manifest themselves depending on weather conditions in the various seasons; wind/*loong* humor imbalances manifest in late summer and in the late evening and overnight; those of bile/*tripa* manifest in the autumn, at noon, and at midnight; and those of phlegm/*beken* in spring, morning, and evening. Similarly, Tibetan doctors give dietary recommendations depending on seasonal weather conditions. At the beginning of summer and winter, hot quality food with sweet, sour, and salty tastes is advised; in spring, rough-quality food with bitter, pungent, and astringent tastes; and in autumn, fresh quality food with sweet, bitter, and astringent tastes.

Tibetan medicine studies the nature of the protective *la* energy, its cyclical motion inside the body, the specific points of the body where this energy is located depending on the day of the lunar calendar and the time, and the treatment of these points.

The *la* energy is a life force coming from the pure energy of the five elements that permeates and creates the human being, giving it strength, stamina, stability, clarity. *La* allows for not only physical, mental, and sexual satisfaction but also a luminous complexion and harmonic development of the body.

This energy, in its intensity and the body area in which it is concentrated, follows a route, changing at different times of the day, week, and month. The changes are related to the lunar cycle. It has a growing phase and then reaches a peak, from which it enters a decreasing phase. The monthly development is different for men and women.

Every day, *la* energy moves in our body in an accurate cycle. You could say that it is protective energy and is like the essence of individual consciousness. In Tibetan medicine it is considered a very important energy, part of the triad "protective energy, vital energy and energy that regulates the duration of life."[1]

Just as a bowl containing garlic retains the odor even after the garlic has been removed, a part of the *la* energy remains after the consciousness has left the body after death. Depending on the type of disease that led to death and the mental state at the time of death, it may happen that the

---

[1] Tib.: *bLa, srog, tshe: bLa*, the essential energy protective of life; *srog*, the vital energy in the body as a manifestation of consciousness; and *tshe*, energy that regulates the life span.

protective *la* energy of some people stay in the house where the deceased lived, affecting the health of family members and those who live there.

Sometimes, due to an imbalance or a lack in energy level, part of the protective energy of the individual may leave the body. The main points through which protective energy can leave are the ring fingers of the hands and the fourth toes of the feet. It can also be removed by the powers or by the influence of elements present in the external environment or other beings.

Due to an injury somewhere in the body where the protective *la* energy is present at any moment, the whole body can suffer severe damage and may be compromised; even life may be threatened. To avoid damaging the protective *la* energy and therefore the body, we tie red strings at the base of the ring fingers and fourth toes when practicing massage to prevent losing the positive energy and absorbing negative energy. Avoid excessively strong pressure on the points where the protective energy is present on the day of treatment. And particularly on those points on those days, never apply moxa or do bloodletting.

La can leave the body due to too vigorous massage; invasive therapies; moxa, acupuncture, and bloodletting in the area where *la* is present; very strong pressure, shocks, traumatic accidents, major surgery, wounds, and bruises.

Symptoms that suggest the partial loss of the protective energy are a feeling of sadness, fatigue, anxiety, dull and grayish skin, obscuration of memory, mental confusion and agitation, and particularly, sudden and repeated awakenings during sleep.

When the protective *la* energy of a person is in good condition, the person is physically well, the body is strong and the mind is clear and happy.

Monthly Cycle of the Protective *La* Energy

The *la* energy moves in the body in a cycle concurrent with the waxing and waning phases of the moon, constellations, and planets and assumes shapes that resemble letters of the Tibetan alphabet. Its movement has three defined phases: active, rising, and dissolving. The active phase is when the protective energy performs its functions in a particular section of the body; on same day, a part of the protective energy is in the dissolving phase at the body point where it was present the day before and

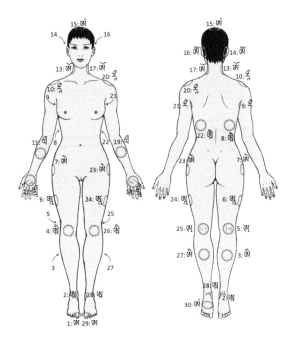

FIG. 45. Monthly circulation of the *la* energy

another part is in the rising phase at the body point where it will be the next day. The *la* energy begins its cyclical movement on the first day of the lunar month. For men it starts from the left foot and for women, from the right foot.

The protective *la* energy moves through two cycles of movements, monthly and daily.

Massage for Rebalancing the Protective Energy *La*

In the tradition of Bon and Buddhism, there are *la* rituals used to "hook" back lost *la* and also to strengthen *la*. Many Buddhist deity and dakini practices are also connected to *la*. In Yuthok Nyingthik's text, there are practices for "hooking" back the *la* through Hayagriva (the wrathful man-ifestation of Avalokiteśvara or Guanyin Bodhisattva) and Dakini practices. However, even without spiritual rituals, we can protect and strengthen the *la*. One very simple way is to wear red thread or rings on the ring fingers and fourth toes to prevent losing the positive energy and absorbing negative energy.

La massage is one of the most effective methods to attract back the dispersed protective energy. The massage is executed in areas where the energy is present at the time, then at the point where it was the day before, and finally where it will pass the following day. Or it may be extended to the entire body, treating every *la* point, tracing lightly with the fingertips, drawing and visualizing the protective energy in the form of the corresponding Tibetan letter surrounded by a light sphere while reciting the appropriate sound. Preparations are used with butter or sesame oil, or oil suitable for the wind/*loong* typology.

Besides receiving *la* massage from a therapist, an individual can do self-massage, gently massaging each *la* point in a circular motion with the palm while reciting the "*Ali*" mantra (vowels of the Sanskrit alphabet: om a ā i ī u ū ri rī li lī e eē o oō am ah) 21 or 101 times.

Massage on the protective *la* energy points increases feelings of well-being, dispels sorrow, helps cases of mental imbalances, rebalances the energy, relaxes, gives longevity, preserves the sperm and the positive energy, and is recognized as very effective in increasing the sexual capacity of the individual.

Conclusion

HERE OUR JOURNEY to Tanadug, the realm of the Medicine Buddha, comes to an end. I hope that you have enjoyed it and found it useful for yourself and others. This is just a glimpse of the richness of Tibetan medical tradition; there is still much more to discover! In the coming books you can learn about the spiritual path of Tibetan medicine, the sacred art of mantra healing, medical dream analysis, Tibetan geomancy (*sa che*), and much more.

My deep wish is that this work helps many people find ultimate balance, on the physical, energetic, and mental levels.

Dr. Nida Chenagtsang

Appendix 1

Herbs, Foods, and Spices
Used for Healing

THE EASILY ACCESSIBLE food substances described below can be used according to the guidelines of Sowa Rigpa to help maintain or restore humoral balance. They are not considered substitutes for specific therapies, but as recommended additions to a healthy lifestyle.

Following a healthy lifestyle—adequate food intake according to individual typology, enough sleep, physical activity, and positive mental attitude—and using appropriate medicines will prevent illness and reduce visits to specialists, diagnostic examinations, and therapies, and save time and money in the long run.

Absinthe/wormwood (*Artemisia absinthium*): Bitter taste. In TTM it is used in steam and herbal baths.

Amaranth (*Amaranthus caudatus*): Sweet and spicy taste with neutral quality. Lowers fever caused by wind/*loong*, facilitates sweating, helps healing of wounds and diminishes itching, cures leukorrhea (vaginal discharge), increases blood and the body constituents. Great for the young because it stimulates development and is restorative. Contraindicated in cases of hypertension or diarrhea.

Angelica, garden (*Angelica archangelica*): Sweet taste and tepid quality. Indicated for disorders of phlegm/*beken* and wind/*loong*, and kidney diseases; increases the blood and body temperature, reduces excess lymphatic liquid, and relieves indigestion and wind diseases. Should not be used in cases of fever, diabetes, or bile/*tripa* pathologies. It is used as an infusion made by putting a cup of crushed roots in a bowl of hot water for 5–10 minutes, or as a decoction.

Asafoetida (*Ferula assafoetida*): Spicy and has the characteristic of heating; increases the digestive fire and so facilitates the assimilation of foods and stimulates the appetite. A good antagonist of the cold afflictions and wind/*loong* imbalances. It also has antibacterial properties.

Bamboo culm (*Bambusa textilis*): A whitish powder found in the stem of the bamboo. Has cool potency and a slightly sweet taste. The best medicine for lung disorders. It has healing properties and is used to treat infected wounds.

Barley (*Hordeum vulgare L.*): Sweet taste and a heavy and cold quality. Increases intestinal peristalsis and so has laxative properties as well as an antihypertensive effect. Also useful as an antiflu medication and to heal urinary infections. Great as a tonic. Cures the diseases of wind/*loong*. When toasted, it acquires the quality of being light; indicated also in cases of phlegm/*beken*.

Buckwheat (*Fagopyrum esculentum*): Astringent and sweet tone, fresh and light quality. Increases the three humors, helps heal wounds, and gives nutriment to the skin.

Butter: Sweet taste, cool quality, purgative. Increases fertility, makes the complexion luminous, eliminates fever that arises due to bile/*tripa* or wind/*loong* imbalances, increases digestive heat.

Buttermilk: Astringent and sour taste, light and hot quality. Stimulates both the appetite and digestive heat. Cures stomach and spleen diseases, helps to reduce edema, and cures hemorrhoids and dysuria (painful or difficult urination).

Camphor (*Cinnamomum camphora*): Derives from the distillation of the bark and wood of *Cinnamomun camphora*. Can be used to eliminate high fever and forms of persistent chronic pyrexia (elevated body temperature). Should be consumed carefully, as it can have toxic effects.

Cardamom (*Elettaria cardamomum*): Its capacity for curing kidney diseases is well known. Treats all cases of cold nature dysfunctions and kidney disorders specifically of cold nature, cases of retention and/or urinary infection, impotence, and decrease in sexual energy and desire. Can be used to flavor food or as a hot infusion.

Cardamom, long (*Amomum subulatum*): Considered the "supreme medicine" to cure stomach and spleen diseases of cold origin, like metabolic and digestive problems.

Celery (*Apium graveolens*): Sweet, spicy tonality and fresh quality. Useful to treat fever, pulmonary diseases, bad feeling after hangover, and thirst; it increases the appetite, develops antiherpetic action, increases stomach heat, eliminates the presence of blood in the urine, cures cystitis and night enuresis. It is an antihypertensive. Not to be used in cases of excess phlegm/*beken*. The seeds are used in infusions; the stalks can be centrifuged and drunk, and can be added raw or cooked in several culinary preparations.

Chamomile (*Matricaria recutita*): Sweet taste. Relaxing, anti-inflammatory, antiallergic. Indicated to pacify the excesses of wind/*loong*.

Chili (*Capsicum*): Spicy taste that heats, properties conferred by the capsaicin, a chemical substance. Increases the digestive heat; of great help to pacify wind/*loong*, hemorrhoids, lymphatic infections, and hydrops. Used in the diet, it helps to burn fat, eliminates bacteria, and prevent tumors and cysts. If consumed in excess, it can cause a burning feeling in the stomach, throat, and lips and weaken energy. Contraindicated for bile/*tripa* typologies, fever, pulmonary infections, ocular infections, bleeding, and gastric problems.

Cinnamon (*Cinnamomum zeylanicum*): The taste is hot, sweet, astringent, and salty, with heating properties. It increases digestive fire, the appetites, giving strength to the body. Reduces cold in the stomach, wind/*loong* afflictions, and liver and pulmonary infectious secretions. For flu and colds, drink half a glass of infusion two to three times during the day. Contraindicated in cases of bile/*tripa* and in hot nature pathologies.

Chickpeas (*Cicer arietinum*): Astringent and sweet taste, fresh potentiality, light and absorbent. Great for the combined wind/*loong*–phlegm/*beken* disorders; eliminates excesses of mucus; useful for asthma; cures hemorrhoids; and eliminates diarrhea and fat.

Cloves (*Caryophyllus aromaticus*): Useful for blood pressure problems that are influenced by wind/*loong*. It is also used to calm panic attacks and depression. Used to flavor food but also as an infusion and can be added to other substances like nutmeg and star anise to calm wind/*loong*. It should be taken hot.

Coriander seed (*Coriandrum sativum*). In Sowa Rigpa, it is considered a superlative medicine. The taste is sweet and spicy. Helps reduce phlegm/*beken* and wind/*loong* disorders, cures gastric problems, and is antipyretic.

Corn (*Zea mays*): Sweet and astringent taste; hot, dry, and light nature. Administer for phlegm/*beken* disorders; facilitates digestion. Useful in cases of gallstones and urinary stones.

Cumin, black (*Bunium bulbocastanum*): Spicy and sweet taste. Has heating properties that heal hepatic problems associated with cold origin (e.g., gallstones). Useful to heal digestive pathologies and in case of flatulence, for it increases the digestive fire and helps in food assimilation. Cntraindicated in the presence of bile/*tripa* disorders.

Cumin, white (*Cuminum cyminum*): The taste is spicy and sweet; cures phlegm/*beken* indigestion and flatulence. Useful in cases of mental disease. The yellow type is useful in pulmonary disease. It should be avoided for high fever and bile/*tripa* disorders.

Dandelion (*Taraxacum officinale*): Sweet and bitter taste, refreshing quality. It is a good antagonist of chronic fevers, epidemics, and intoxication and helps overcome gastroenteritis. Has properties that helps remove toxins in the stomach and the gall bladder. Using the leaves in salads will help to prevent and eventually heal gallstones. The root in the form of infusion has a purifying effect in the hepatic parenchyma, stimulating bile production. The diuretic action produces an antihypertensive effect.

Eggplant (*Solanum melongena*): Sweet taste and lightly cooling characteristics that make it a great antagonist against blood and heat disorders. Gives relief of ulcerative colitis and skin infections, improves anuria, lowers blood pressure. Contraindicated in people with chronic diarrhea and weak digestive force.

Fennel seed (*Foeniculum vulgare*): Sweet and slightly spicy taste. Increases digestive temperature and the physical constituents, has carminative (antigas) properties, eliminates hiccups, helps in the assimilation of foods, helps appetite, reduces intestinal bacteria, cleans the breath, and promotes diuresis. Can be eaten raw or cooked. Indicated for the preparation of good herbal teas, particularly after a heavy meal. Should be used with caution during pregnancy, in the presence of bile/*tripa* disorders, and in cases of abundant menstruation.

Garlic (*Allium sativum*): Has a spicy taste and heat nature. Calms the wind/*loong* excesses; relieves abdominal cramps, bacterial infections, colds, flu, and water retention; reduces cholesterol, thins the blood, and has antihypertensive action. It is an intestinal antiparasitic, induces relaxation, reduces intoxication effects, and increases the body temperature, the digestive heat, and the appetite. Used to give flavor to foods.

Ghee (*clarified butter*): Sweet taste and hot quality. Reinforces the metabolic heat, strengthens the body, and sharpens the mind in times of mental fatigue.

Ginger (*Zingiber officinale*): A well-known and appreciated plant in the West and East, for its curative capacities. Has a spicy taste and a heating quality. Sowa Rigpa uses three base varieties and many other secondary varieties that have similar functions; increases digestion and heats the body due to the presence of the gingerol molecules. The root is used in the preparation of more than fifty medicines. Five varieties that can be obtained easily:

> *Ginger decoction:* The more simple way of use. Add a teaspoon of macerated dry or fresh ginger to two cups of water and boil slowly, until the liquid is reduced by half. Should be drunk hot and can be used in cases of indigestion, slow digestion, cold sensation in the body or cold hands and feet, fatigue, or drowsiness.

> *Decoction of rock salt:* Ingredients required: rock salt (Tibetan salt), ginger, and arura (*Terminalia chebula*). Use the same quantity of salt and ginger, and half that amount of arura. Introduce the three ingredients in cold water, bringing everything to a boil for a short period of time. Drink the preparation hot. Indicated for cold origin disorders, cold sensation in the articulations, hypotension, and indigestion.

> *Tisane of the three substances:* 100 grams of ginger, 100 grams of asafetida (*Ferula asafoetida*), and 5 grams of salt (*Halitum violaceum*). Mix tand add a spoonful of this compound to a glass of hot water; drink the preparation hot. Indicated in cases of insomnia, emotional instability, sadness, depression (excess wind/*loong* at the heart level).

> *Infusion of the three hot herbs:* Black pepper, ginger, and long pepper in equal parts. Add to hot water and boil until two thirds of the liquid evaporates. Advisable for imbalances caused by cold, particularly in wind/*loong* disorders with symptoms like chills, tremors, cold in the extremities, emotional and mental instability, headaches with a cold feeling, indigestion.

Ginger single formula: Put a thin slice of fresh ginger on the tongue for five to ten minutes. Used for swelling and pimples on the tongue.

Honey: Sweet taste and hot quality. Has a toning effect, increases the digestive heat, useful in phlegm/*beken* disorders.

Kidney bean (*Phaseolus vulgaris*): Sweet taste, fresh and heavy characteristics. Cures wind/*loong* diseases, increases phlegm/*beken* and bile/*tripa* energy.

Lemon (*Citrus limonum*): Sour and astringent taste. Increases heat, stimulates the appetite, and improves digestion. Water with lemon juice can be drunk to aid in the assimilation of an abundant meal. It has antiseptic and depurative properties and can be used diluted as a gargle in cases of disorders of the throat. Diluted juice with cinnamon and garlic infusion, taken hot, can be useful to cure colds and flu.

Lentils (*Lens culinaris*): Astringent and sweet taste, fresh quality, light and absorbent. Increases the three humors and cures hemorrhoids. Externally used as mask; cures gout, erysipelas, and hypertension.

Licorice (*Glycyrrhiza glabra*): The root, harvested in autumn, has a sweet taste and cures wind/*loong* and channels disorders. It should be used in the form of decoction, to cure colds and indigestions. Has expectorant properties, diminishes cough, and calms asthma. Has anti-inflammatory properties for arthritic articulations. It is a good medicine for liver problems by pacifying wind/*loong*. Has a hypertensive action.

Linseed (*Linum usitatissimum*): Sweet taste, bitter character, oily and soft. Useful for wind/*loong* disorders. If used with milk, induces sleep and relaxation. The golden type can be used regularly.

Lotus root (*Nelumbo nucifera*): Sweet-astringent tonic; reinforces the body constituents, increases skin luminosity, and lowers fever. Used for blood loss and to fight insomnia. Contraindicated for those with weak digestive heat, diarrhea, and stomach cramps.

Mallow (*Malva sylvestris*): Has a sweet taste and cooling quality; reinforces the kidneys, gives relief from kidney inflammation and to the bladder. Useful in cases of urinary retention and diarrhea, and quenches thirst. Drains complicated wounds of pus and serum. The leaves and stems are used, fried, cooked in soup, and also eaten in salads. Should not be used if there is an excess of phlegm/*beken* or in cold disorders.

Millet (*Panicum miliaceum*): Sweet taste, heavy and fresh quality. Stimulates growth, has tonic properties, helps fracture calcification, cures wind/*loong* and bile/*tripa* disorders, increases phlegm/*beken*.

Mustard: Astringent and spicy taste. Indicated to drain blood impurities and lymphatic fluids. Useful in the treatment of inflammations, as mucolytic in pulmonary infections, and to reduce swelling in cases of fluid retention. Contraindicated in the presence of enlargement of the spleen.

Nettle (*Utica dioica*): Sweet-spiced tonality with the tendency to heat. Provides heat, helps in food assimilation, useful in indigestion caused by vegetables, reinforces the organism. Calms wind excesses. Useful for diuresis in the cure of external hemorrhage, for abundant menstrual cycles, and for anemic states. It can be used in decoction from the roots or as infusion from the leaves. Contraindicated in cases of excess phlegm/*beken*–bile/*tripa*, hypertension, and imbalances of a hot origin.

Nutmeg (*Myristica fragans*): A heart tonic. According to the *Four Tantras*, it is indicated to calm disorders due to excess wind/*loong* by restoring circulation. Used mainly to eradicate all problems of this energy and also the one in the heart (*Nying loong*). In Tibetan medicine, "heart problems" are either cardiovascular functions or connected to the emotions. *Nying loong* regulates the senses, the perceptions, and the emotions and is located in the heart. Nutmeg is added to culinary dishes to impart flavor and used isolated to make tisanes, or used with other spices that serve to regulate wind/*loong* disorders. Do not overdose, as it can have a hallucinogenic effect.

Olive oil (*Olea europaea*): Hot taste and heavy quality. Functions as a hepatic purifier.

Onion (*Allium cepa*): Spicy, develops heat. Increases the digestive fire, induces sleep. Eliminates wind/*loong* and phlegm/*beken* excesses, reduces inveterate edema, increases vitality, stops bleeding, and, if regularly used, protects against colon cancer. Contraindicated for bile/*tripa* typology, in case of fever, and in persons with pungent body odor or who sweat a lot.

Parthenium/Feverfew (*Parthenium hysterophorus*): Has a vasodilator action and therefore is useful in the treatment of vasomotor headache. Used with other herbs as analgesic and in cases of arthritis. An anti-coagulant; avoid during pregnancy.

Pepper, black (*Piper nigrum*): Obtained from a vine plant that can grow up to six meters in height and starts to produce fruit between the second and fifth year. It is produced due to the fermentation process caused by fungus that reaches the immature fruits. Has a hot taste and heating properties from a substance called piperina. A good antagonist of phlegm/*beken* and cold imbalances and in cases of food intoxication. Good for digestive heat; calms stomach problems and menstruation problems caused by cold origin pathologies. Induces an increase in body temperature. Too much can increase fever, bile/*tripa* humor, thirst, and hot origin infections.

Pepper, long (*Piper longum*): Hot taste and heating faculties. Indicated to renew weak digestive fire; alleviates phlegm/*beken* and wind/*loong* disorders, respiratory problems, indigestion, and flatulence. Also useful for invigorating renal heat and in cases of sexual impotency. Can aggravate febrile states and gastric problems.

Peppermint (*Mentha piperita*): A taste that is transformed from astringent to hot and characteristics that vary from hot to pleasantly fresh. Increases digestive fire; stimulates the appetite; relieves fever caused by wind/*loong*, ulcers, and eruptions; and calms muscular pains. Also useful in throat infections and for swelling of the eyelids. The leaves can be used to flavor dishes, in salads, or in infusions or added to tea.

Pomegranate (*Punica granatum*): Astringent and sweet taste, hot nature. Cures wind/*loong* disorders, increases digestive heat, and cures stomach infections of cold origin and excesses of phlegm/*beken*. Also stimulates the appetite and calms diarrhea caused by cold. Sowa Rigpa uses all parts of the fruit, also in powder form. Squeeze the fruit fresh, or use the seeds to add an exotic touch to foods.

Rice (*Oryza sativa*): Sweet taste, oily and soft quality. Fresh and light, it allows the elimination of the three humor disorders, dissipates vomiting and diarrhea, and increases fertility.

Saffron (*Crocus sativus*): Very effective in the form of tisane, to heal the liver and bile. Useful for healing bleeding (gastric ulcers, excessively abundant menstruation, bleeding of external wounds). Antipyretic; stimulates the immune system. Can help increase concentration. For a tisane, put a pinch of powdered saffron into a cup of boiling water; leave to rest for ten minutes before drinking. Can also be used as a decoction: put 5 grams in a liter of cold water, bring to boil for about ten minutes. Drink the decoction sweetened with honey. Do not extend the boiling time, as it can acquire a bitter taste. Can be prepared in a compound tisane with other spices like clove, cinnamon, and star anise. Can be used in culinary preparations, either sweetened or salted.

Salt (*Halit*): Salty taste and hot properties. Stimulates the appetite, increases digestive fire, increases the breakdown of foods, regulates intestinal movement, and helps to eliminate wastes. Useful in wind/*loong* imbalance. If consumed in excessive doses, increases bile/*tripa* and causes hypertension, hair loss, hair whitening, skin aging, and damage to the eyes.

Salvia (*Salvia officinalis*): Moderately bitter taste; can be used as antiseptic in cases of sore throat, gingivitis, and thrush. Useful for calming irritations caused by insect bites; helps digestion and stimulates the nervous system. Also useful for regulating menstrual flow. The infusion calms a sore throat.

Sandalwood, red (*Pterocarpus santalinus*): The tree from which it is extracted has a red trunk and green leaves. Used in cases of herpetic infections, hypertension, and pain in the upper back (wind/*loong* zone). Applied externally in pomade, cures articular swelling.

Sandalwood, white (*Santalum album*): The tree has a white trunk and green leaves. Used to heal infections caused by pulmonary pathologies, cardiac diseases, and intermittent fever. The fragrance improves sensorial perception, reduces drowsiness, and induces mental clarity.

Sesame oil (*Sesamum indicum*): Sweet taste, hot and sharp strength. Stimulates weight loss, tones muscle tissue, and reinforces the body. Indicated in wind/*loong*–phlegm/*beken* disorders. Can be used as a condiment and in culinary preparations, and applied externally as a massage oil.

Sesame seeds (*Sesamum indicum*): Sweet tonality, heavy and hot properties. Cures wind/*loong* disorders, has aphrodisiac properties, and increases fertility.

Soybean (*Glycine max*): Sweet taste and neutral properties. Increases the body constituents, diminishes wind/*loong*, combats the effects of intoxication, has a good diuretic effect, and reduces water retention.

Star anise (*Illicium verum*): Hot and sweet taste; increases heat. Pacifies stomach cramps; eliminates flatulence, anuria, constipation, and kidney pains. Contraindicated for bile/*tripa* cases, hot infections, and cases of fever with thirst.

Sugar cane (*Saccharum spp.*): Sweet taste and cooling properties. Useful for wind/*loong* conditions; the sugar cane normalizes the excess. Also helpful for nausea and bile disorders. To be avoided by the phlegm/*beken* typology.

Sunflower seed oil (*Helianthus annuus*): Sweet quality and hot strength. Cold-pressed sunflower seed oil is an emollient and sebum regulator rich in vitamin E. Useful for the treatment of chapped, dry, dehydrated, and sensitive skin. Useful for the wind/*loong* pathologies. Used as a condiment and in culinary preparations, and applied externally as a massage oil.

Turmeric (*Curcuma longa*): Spicy and bitter taste and fresh quality. Indicated in cases of intoxication, infection, and hemorrhoid infection. Regulates bile flow. Can be used to improve digestion, to lower fever in cases of dysentery, for arthritis, in hepatic disorder, to calm menstrual cramps, and to reduce flatulence, blood in the urine, and very high levels of cholesterol in the blood. Can be used in powder, as mother tincture, or as essential oil. Great as herbal tea or in food preparation. Use cautiously in cases of gallstones; avoid use in pregnancy and during lactation.

Wheat (*Triticum sp.*): Sweet taste that transforms into astringent and heavy quality, fresh and nutritive. Helps in the elimination of wind/*loong* and bile/*tripa* disorders. If used in modest quantities and on alternate days, rebalances the three humors. Not advisable in cases of phlegm/*beken* increasing. Natural organic wild wheat such as einkorn, spelt, emmer, or kamut should be used, not the genetically modified types, as the tastes and qualities are altered.

Zucchini (*Cucurbita pepo*): Taste from sweet to bitter; lightly refreshing property. Reinforces the body constituents, increases a mother's milk flow, and also has a bactericidal action.

Appendix 2

History of *Yukchö*, Stick Massage

MASSAGE WITH STICKS is said to have developed in two different ways: through combined medical and spiritual practice and through research and experience related exclusively to the medical field.

The first written record was found in the *terma*[1] rediscovered by Rat-nalingpa[2] called *Massage with Stick, the Secret Union of Jewels That Satisfies Desires*, presented as a tool for yogis to overcome their physical problems, for use after reciting the mantra of a specific deity. The same mantra was also used to enhance the mustard seeds (by blowing on them) used to fill small cloth pouches, traditionally placed on the tip of the stick, to soften the tapping. This type of massage was introduced by tantric yogis, disciples of the spiritual tradition of the secular Ngakpas, founded in the eighth century by Padmasambhava, which conferred powers and blessings through instruments such as the ritual triangular lamina dagger (*phurba*), ritual linen handkerchief (*bakhar*), trumpet made from a femur (*kangdung*), and vajra (*dorje*). Stick massage is deeply connected with

---

[1] Terma (*gter ma*): teachings or objects hidden by a spiritual leader to be rediscovered in a successive period by the predestined person.

[2] A great Tibetan religious figure of the fifteenth century.

spiritual practice and with Ratnalingpa, and therefore was performed only by yogis.

A second theory holds that stick massage could have evolved independently and later been incorporated into religious practice. The text *The Instructions on Massage with the Stick That Has a Diamond Quality* by Dr. Gyaltsen Pelzang presented this technique as a medical practice, using visualizations of nonreligious nature and belonging exclusively to the medical system.

Stick massage likely originated from primitive people's efforts to ease pain in the upper back by hitting with a fist or pressing with an elbow. During the Palaeolithic and Neolithic periods, when men began to use stone and wood instruments to meet the demands of everyday life, the method of using a stick with a round stone attached to its end was born. Due to accumulated experiences over the centuries, stick massage is now considered a medical therapy.

In any case, if there were no historical basis for this practice, long and detailed texts would not have been written and survived until now. It is evident that the stick massage technique is uniquely Tibetan, not imported from other countries.

Apart from some specific features that characterize the stick massage found in religious practice, such as the chanting of mantras and visualization of a deity, the main practice of stick massage is essentially identical in the religious and medical traditions. Both books described how to do the massage, the points to be focused on, indications, and contraindications with the same details.

The practice of stick massage was suspended in Tibet for a very long time, due to the fact that in most cases, the therapy must be repeated many times over a short period to be effective. This constituted a major obstacle for the Tibetans, who have lived and still live in secluded places very distant from each other. Even today, travel is difficult, and most of the inhabitants can receive treatment from a doctor only after a few days away from home.

Therapies such as moxibustion and cupping were easier to implement and produced therapeutic results more quickly. For all these reasons, Tibetan doctors naturally used them in place of stick massage. Moreover, most modern doctors do not have a deep interest in ancient healing external therapies and heal patients using drugs alone. For the same reason, the tradition of minor surgery has been almost completely lost in Tibet.

The only operation that is practiced today is for cataracts, and there are very few doctors who are able to do so. The same is true of acupuncture according to Tibetan tradition. Probably this was the real cause of the gradual abandonment of minor surgical operations and stick massage.

These therapies have always been surrounded by an aura of secrecy and often transmitted to a single student at a time. Secrecy has also partly contributed to their decline. For example, the content of *The Instructions on Massage with the Stick That Has a Diamond Quality* was passed down orally and continuously until the time of Dr. Gyaltsen Pelzang, who first put it in writing in a technical book, written for the benefit of others "by request of the disciples in question."

The most important books on stick massage that this research is based upon are:

Massage with Stick, the Secret Union of Jewels That Satisfies Desires, a *terma* of Ratna Lingpa extracted from the collection called "The Treasure of the Precious Termas"[3] by Jamgon Kongtrul (1811–99)

The Instructions on Massage with the Stick That Has a Diamond Quality by Gyaltsen Pelzang, discovered in the Potala Library in Lhasa.

Instructions on Massage with the Stick That Has a Diamond Quality or *The Arrow of Meteoric Iron That Strikes Every Disease and Provocation* by Deumar Tenzin, nineteenth century.

---

[3] *Rin chen gter mdzod.*

Glossary

These are the Tibetan terms used in the book, with English pronunciation. They are placed in alphabetical order, with a Wylie transliteration and an English translation.

PHONETIC	WYLIE TRANSLITERATION	ENGLISH TRANSLATION
bakhar	sba 'khar	ritual linen handkerchief
beken	badkan	phlegm humor; literally "water and earth"
Bigje	'bigs byed, Skt. Vindhya	Thunderbolt or "Penetrative" Mountain in the southern garden of Tanadug with the strength and power of the sun
buguchen	sbugucan	tubular channel
bum shi	'bum bzhi	ancient treatise on Tibetan medicine, *The Four Thousand Ways of Medicine*, containing transcripts of medical teachings of Bon Master Sherab Miwoche, written by his son Chebu Trise
chag	lcag	metal
chang	chang	Tibetan drink made from fermented wheat, barley, or rice
Chebu Trise	dpyat bu khri shes	first Tibetan doctor, son of Bon Master Sherab Miwoche

chima gyu	phyi ma rgyud	Final Tantra or Tantra of Final Action
cho	chos, Skt. dharma	dharma; phenomenon
cho	cos	heart chakra; dharma of phenomenon
chu	chu	water
chu me	chu me	water moxa
chug pa	byug pa	massage, oil application
chulum	chulums	bath therapy
dang gyur tripa	mdangs sgyur mkhris pa	color-producing bile
dangma	dangs ma	nutritional essence
dechen	bde chen	head chakra; great bliss
dekyong	bde skyong	base chakra; pleasure
dewa	bde ba	happiness
dhochag	'dod chags	attachment, desire
do nye	rdo mnye	massage with stone
död yönten nga	'dod yon tan nga	the knowledge of desire that manifests through the senses
dok sel tripa	mdog gsal mkhris pa	complexion-clearing bile
don	gdon	negative influences or external provocations
dorje	rdo rje	vajra
drangwa	grangwa	cold nature condition related to wind and phlegm
drubje tripa	sgrub byed mkhris pa	energizing bile; bile of desire, ego
dud	ndud	black spirits
dug sum	dug gsum	three mental poisons: attachment, anger, ignorance
dutsi nga lum	bdud rtsi lnga lums	five-nectar bath
Gangcen	gangs can, Skt. Himavata	"Snow-capped" Mountain in the northern part of Tanadug, imbued with lunar qualities
gen gyu loong	gyen rgyu rlung	ascending wind
gyud shi	rgyud bzhi	the four medical tantras
horme	horme	Mongolian hot oil moxibustion
ja che	'ja byed	channels of paralysis
jorje beken	'byor byed bad kan	connective phlegm
Ju Mipam Gyatso	'ju mi pham rgya mtsho	one of the greatest Tibetan scholars of philosophy, astrology, and medicine of the nineteenth century; author of fourteen texts; famous for his personal style in the preparation of remedies
juje tripa	'ju byed mkhris pa	digestive bile
jung va	'byung ba	elements of origin

jung va nga	'byung ba lnga	five internal elements
kam nye	skam mnye	dry massage without the use of oils
kang	rkang	bone marrow
kangdung	rkang dung	ritual trumpet
kham	khams	external energies
kham nga	khams lnga	five external elements
khil khor	dkyil 'khor, Skt. maṇḍala	mandala; a symbol representing perfect balance with one center and four directions
khorlo	'khor lo	chakra; branching center of channels and energy in the body
khyab je loong	khyab byed rlung	all-pervasive wind
kunye	bsku mnye, bku mnye	Tibetan massage
kuwa	khu ba	reproductive fluids
kyang ma	rkyang ma	left lunar channel
la	bLa	protective supreme energy that moves and resides on specific sites of the body according to the moon cycles
lagtong	lhag mthong, Skt. vipaśyanā	analytical meditation, vipassana
ley loong	las rlung	karmic wind
lon nye	rlon mnye	massage with the use of oils
long cho	longs spyod	throat chakra; joy or experience
loong	rLung	wind humor; translated as wind or air, although an older meaning is movement
loong dug	rlung du	smoke therapy; fumigation
loong sem	rlung sems	fusion of wind and mind
lotsawa	lo tsa ba	translator; referring to the great translator Marpa
Malaya	ma la ya	"Garlanded" Mountain in the west of Tanadug containing the six good substances, five types of calcites, mineral exudates, mineral waters, and hot springs that pacify all diseases
me	me	fire
me bum	me bum	literally "vase of fire"; cupping
me sang	me gsang	moxa points
Men ngak gyu	man ngag rgyud	Oral Instruction Tantra
Mentsee khang	sman rtsis khang	Tibetan Medical and Astrological Institute
menyam loong	me mnyam rlung	wind that assists digestive heat
metsa	me btsa	moxibustion
Milarepa	mi la res pa	Tibet's most famous yogi, heart disciple of Marpa, foremost student of Naropa

nága	klu, Skt. nāga	serpent spirit
namkha	nam mkha	space
ne mey	nad med	good health
nejang	gnas sbyangs	Tibetan healing yoga
ngab ra	ngab grwa	sucking horn used in horn therapy
ngakpa	ngag pa	Tibetan yogis
nor	nor	wealth
nyak je beken	myag byed bad kan	mixing phlegm
nyepa	nyes pa	literally "faults," referring to the imbalanced state of the three humors
nying loong	rnying rlung	wind in the heart
nyong je beken	myong byed bad kan	tasting phlegm
phurba	phur ba	ritual dagger
Pöngaden	spos ngad ldan	"Fragrant" Mountain in the east of Tanadug where grows a forest of arura trees
ra tsug	grwa tshug	moxa with horn
rag loong	rag rlung	coarse or gross wind
rag pa	rags pa	gross, coarse aspect of element
ratna	ratna	precious
Ratna Lingpa	ratna gling pa	a great Tibetan religious figure of the fifteen century
Rigpe Yeley Kye	rigs pa'i yid las skye	emanation of the speech of Buddha
Rigpe Yeshe	rigs pa'i ye shes	emanation of the mind of Buddha
Rinchen terdzö	rin chen gter mdzod	"The Treasure of the Precious Termas"
roma	roma	right solar channel
rü	rus	bone
sa	sa	earth
Sangye Menla	sangs rgyas sman bla	*sang*, awake; *gye*, developed five wisdoms; *men*, medicine; *la*, guru; Medicine Buddha
sha	sha	muscle tissue
she dang	zhe sdang	anger, hatred, aversion
She gyu	bshad rgyud	Explanatory Tantra
Sherab Miwoche	gshen rab mi bo che	Tibetan Bon master
shiney	zhi gnas, Skt. samatha	calm abiding mind
shing	shing	wood
shing tsug	shing tshug	moxa with wood
sogzin loong	srog dzin rlung	life-sustaining wind
sowa	sro ba	heating; third part of *ku* massage

Sowa Rigpa	gso ba rigs pa	literally "Healing Science"; vernacular name of Traditional Tibetan Medicine
Tanadug	lta na sdug	literally "pleasing when looked upon"; pure land or garden of the Medicine Buddha
tar sang	gtar gsang	bloodletting points
telme	telme	moxa with metal
ten je beken	rten byed bad kan	supporting phlegm
terma	gter ma	literally "hidden treasure"; refers to secret spiritual teachings hidden away by Guru Rinpoche or his consort Yeshe Tsogyal in the eighth century to be discovered in the future by so-called *tertön*s (treasure revealers)
thangka	thang ka	sacred Tibetan scroll painting usually depicting a Buddhist deity, scene, or mandala
thongje tripa	mthong byed mkhris pa	vision-producing bile
thur sang	thur gsang	acupuncture points
thur sel loong	thur sel rlung	descending wind
timook	gti mug	ignorance, delusion
tra loong	phra rlung	subtle wind
trag	khrag	blood
trawa	phra ba	subtle aspect of element
tripa	mkhrispa	bile humor; means fire or burn
trul pai	trum pa'i	navel chakra; manifestation or emanation
tsa dud	rtsa sdud	knots where the channels meet; connected to the five elements and the origin of chakras
tsa gyu	rtsa rgyud	Root Tantra
tsakhor	rtsa 'khor	channel and wheel; wheels formed by channels, referring to the chakras
tsang bug	tshang bug	crown point
tsawa	tsawa	hot nature condition related to blood and bile
tsawa sum	rtsa ba gsum	three roots; referring to the Three Trees of TTM
tsering	tshe ring	long life
tsig jor	tshig sbyor	joint mobilization
tsil	tshil	adipose tissue; fat
tsim je beken	tsim byed bad kan	satisfying phlegm
tummo	gtum mo	divine fire yoga
uma	uma	central channel
yidam	yi dam, Skt. Istadeva	a buddha as personal object of one's practice

yukchö	dbyug bcos	stick massage
yuk sang	dbyug gsang	points for stick massage
Yuthok Yönten Gönpo	g.yu thog yon tan dgon po	father/founder of Tibetan medicine; author of the *Four Tantras*

Bibliography

Anonymous (ninth century). *Tun hong nas thon pa'i bod kyi gso rig yig cha bdam sgrigs*. Ed. Luo Bingfen, Huang Bufan. Peking: Mi rigs dpe skrun khang, 1983.

Bod ljongs sman rtsis khang gso rig zhib 'jug khang, bLo bzang bstan 'dzin. *gSo rig snying bsdus skya rengs gsar pa*. Lhasa: Bod ljongs mi dmangs dpe skrun khang, 1985.

bsTan 'dzin phun tshogs. "rDo rje dbyug pa'i man ngag nad gdon kun 'joms gnam lcags thog mda'." In *De'u dmar gso rig gces btus*. TBRC W2DB13637. 2: 343–360. Peking: Mi rigs dpe skrun khang, 2007.

dBang 'dus. *Bod gangs can pa'i gso ba rig pa'i dpal ldan rgyud bzhi sogs kyi brda dang dka' gnad 'ga' zhig bkrol ba sngon byon mkhas pa'i gsung rgyun g.yu thog dgongs rgyan zhes bya ba bzhugs so dbang 'dus*. Peking: Mi rigs dpe skrun khang, 1983.

dPyad bu khri shes. *gSo rig 'bum bzhi*. TBRC W1GS4. 1 vol. Peking: Mi rigs dpe skrun khang, 2006. http://tbrc.org/link?RID=W1GS4.

'Jam mgon kong sprul blo gros mtha' yas. "gSang ba 'dus pa'i dbyug bcos yid bzhin nor bu." In *Rin chen gter mdzod chen mo*. TBRC W20578. 73: 302–310. Paro: Ngodrup and Sherab Drimay, 1976–80.

Khro ru tshe rnam. *gSo rig rgyud bzhi'i 'grel chen drang srong zhal lung*. Cheng-tu: Si khron mi rigs dpe skrun khang, 2001.

Legs pa dpal bzang. *rDo rje gsum gyi bsnyen sgrub kyis dbyug bcos rin po che*. TBRC W1KG17146. 1 vols. [s.l.]: [s.n.], [n.d.].

Mi pham rgya mtsho. *mKhyud spyad sna tshogs phyogs bsdus tsinta ma ṇi.* TBRC
W1KG3708. 1 vol. Dharmasala, H.P.: Library of Tibetan Works and Archives,
1985.

Mi pham rgya mtsho. *sMan yig phyogs bsgrigs.* TBRC W30528. 1 vol. Čcheng-tu: Si
khron mi rigs dpe skrun khang, 1992.

Mnyam nyid rdo rje. "Ratna manggas mdzad pa'i dbyug bcos nad gdon kun sel
(85)." In *Man ngag bye ba ring bsrel.* TBRC W29481.: 502–507. Peking: Mi rigs
dpe skrun khang, 2005.

Padma 'byung gnas. "gSang ba 'dus pa'i dbyug bcos yid bzhin nor bu." In *sLob
dpon pad 'byung gi sman yig gces btus.* TBRC W1GS10.: 439–444. Peking: Mi
rigs dpe skrun khang, 2006.

Rin chen 'od zer. *bDud rtsi snying po yan lag brgyad pa gsang ba man ngag gi
rgyud las rtsa rgyud dang bshad rgyud kyi 'grel pa.* Cheng-tu: Si khron mi rigs
dpe skrun khang, 2001.

Roerich, George N. *The Blue Annals.* 1949–53; reprint, Delhi: Motilal Banarsidass,
1996.

Tibetan Buddhist Resource Center. www.tbrc.org.

Tshe dbang. "dbYug bcos gnam lcags rdo rje (27)." In *Tshe dbang brgya rtsa.*
TBRC W2DB4622. : 210–211. Peking: Mi rigs dpe skrun khang, 2007.

Wylie, Turrell V. "A Standard System of Tibetan Transcription." *Harvard Journal
of Asiatic Studies* 22 (1959): 261–267.

Yon tan mgon po. *g.Yu thog snying thig. Bod kyi gso ba rig pa'i gna' dpe phyogs
bsgrigs dpe tshogs.* Peking: Mi rigs dpe skrun khang, 2007.

Yon tan mgon po, a Lung rigs bstan dar. *g.Yu thog pa'i shog dril. rGyud bzhi'i
mtha' dpyod.* TBRC W1KG14626. 1 vol. Peking: Mi rigs dpe skrun khang,
2008.

About Dr. Nida Chenagtsang

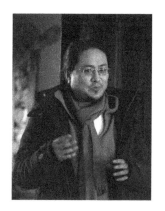

DR. NIDA CHENAGTSANG was born in Amdo, northeastern Tibet. Interested in the traditional healing science of his people, he began his medical studies at the local Traditional Tibetan Medicine hospital. Later he received a scholarship to Lhasa Tibetan Medical University, where he completed his medical education in 1996. Dr Nida completed his practical training at the Traditional Tibetan Medicine hospitals in Lhasa (Lhasa Mentsekhang) and Lhoka.

Dr. Nida has published a number of articles and several books on Traditional Tibetan Medicine. He has extensively researched ancient Tibetan medicinal treatments, specializing in the revival of external therapies, which has brought him high acclaim in the field of Tibetan medicine in both the East and the West. Dr. Nida is the Medical Director of Sorig Khang International (SKI), formerly known as the Academy for Traditional Tibetan Medicine (IATTM), and the Co-Founder of International Ngak-Mang Institutes (NMI), established to preserve and maintain the Rebkong Ngakpa culture within modern Tibetan society.

Dr. Nida's teachings are widely known throughout Asia, Europe, America, and Australia, where he has trained students in Traditional Tibetan Medicine, *kunye* massage, mantra healing, diet and behavior, dream analysis, and *sa che* (geomancy), as well as birth and death according to Tibetan medicine.

About SKI

Facing the imminent loss of Tibetan culture, philosophy, literature, science, and religion, the Sorig Khang International Foundation is to be contributing to the preservation and propagation of Traditional Tibetan Medicine. In particular, the continuity of the holistic Tibetan healing sciences in their theory and their practice, as well as in their philosophy, and in its closely connected spirituality as a complete system in the Yuthok Nyingthig transmission lineage, is to be protected.

— *From the Sorig Khang International Foundation Charter*

THE INTERNATIONAL ACADEMY for Traditional Tibetan Medicine was established by Dr. Nida Chenagtsang in 2006 to ensure the integrity and authenticity of *Sowa Rigpa*—Traditional Tibetan Medicine teachings— and to promote the continuity of its practice. IATTM was officially established as Sorig Khang International (SKI), an international nonprofit foundation based in Germany.

Sowa Rigpa is a holistic system, meaning that it addresses the individual's needs as a whole—body, mind, and spirit—in an integrated way. This includes the individual's internal environment as well as interactions with the external environment. Sowa Rigpa has the capacity to be of great benefit to all in the current economic and social climate.

It is the sincere wish of SKI to keep the spirit of Sowa Rigpa alive and functioning effectively in the modern world. The main aim is to provide courses and training of the highest standard possible, as well as accurate, up-to-date information on Sowa Rigpa as it is currently practiced.

The activities of SKI are organized into five major branches:

1. Providing medical education and spiritual practice
2. Producing and distributing texts and materials
3. Offering connection and support for our international networks of centers, practitioners, teachers, and students
4. Conducting medical and charitable activities
5. Administering our organization.

Through these activities, we share the rich tradition of medical knowledge, healing treatment, and spiritual wisdom offered by Yuthok Yönten Gönpo, the father of Tibetan medicine, with the wish that beings everywhere may experience the fruits of a healthy body and nourished mind.

Find out more about SKI on www.sorig.net!